The Journey Towards Freedom

Quit Alcohol Addiction, Find your True Self,

Discover Happiness and Live Your Dream Life

By

Daniel Mckowen

Table of Contents

Chapter 1: Alcoholism – An Introduction

Human beings had discovered before recorded history that grape juice becomes wine when exposed to naturally occurring yeasts. In the end, scientists would describe this cycle as fermentation, thousands of years after wine and other alcoholic beverages had become an integral part of the meals, festivities and religious ceremonies of many cultures.

Alcoholic beverages sadly have led to a significant portion of human misery. Data from the National Center for Health Statistics indicate that excessive alcohol consumption in the United States alone causes more than 100,000 deaths per year, primarily through liver cirrhosis, drunk driving and alcohol-related homicide and suicide. According to The Columbia University College of Physicists and Surgeons Complete Home Medical Guide, drug use is involved in half of all homicides, accidental deaths and suicides; half of all crimes; and nearly half of all fatal accidents in vehicles.

Nevertheless, the most often associated problem with heavy drinking is alcoholism. In simple words, alcoholism is an addiction to alcohol, but the signs of alcoholism can be difficult to identify beyond this basic definition. They include a desire for alcohol, lack of self-control when drinking, high tolerance for the effects of alcohol, and symptoms of physical withdrawal, such as sweating, shakiness, and anxiety, if alcohol consumption ceases. Alcoholics often continue to drink despite repeated problems associated with alcohol, such as losing a job, harming friends or family, or getting into trouble with the law.

For America alone, there are around 14 million individuals with alcohol problems, of whom just under half are alcoholics. Such estimates are very rough, since many people who drink heavily do not develop the physical and psychological alcohol dependence that characterizes true alcoholics. The terms "drinking problem" or "alcohol abuse" are used to describe these patterns of drinking, which may not lead to alcoholism but are nevertheless often destructive to both drinkers and others.

In fact, nine out of ten drinking people do not become alcoholics. Researchers give many explanations as to why some people seem to be prone to alcoholism, while others are able to drink responsibly — or even abuse alcohol habitually — without becoming dependent upon it. Yet the exact mechanisms behind alcoholism remain poorly understood, despite decades of research. Most scientists agree that there is at least some genetic basis for alcoholism, but they are also quick to warn that biology is only part of the problem. Psychologists point out that while alcoholism tends to run in families, it can be because their parents are learning harmful drinking behaviors. Some researchers point to cultural influences, arguing that people from certain social, racial or socioeconomic backgrounds are more vulnerable than others to alcoholism.

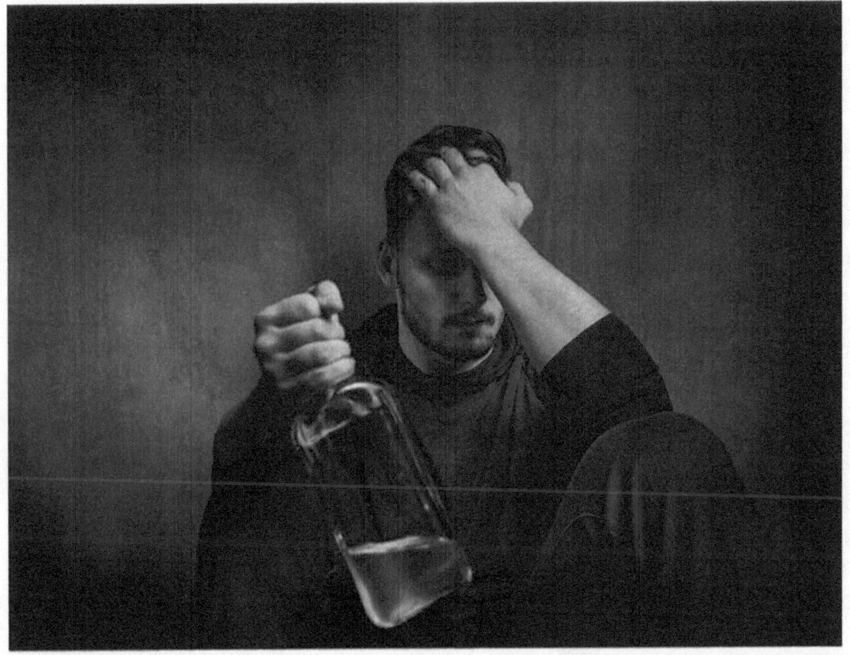

However, the controversy over the causes of alcoholism is a relatively recent phenomenon: until 1860, the term "alcoholism" itself was not coined, and the theory that it is a medical disease was postulated only in 1930. Historically, the debate over compulsive drinking has not been about what induces it, but rather how it can be prevented; those most concerned with alcoholism have not attempted to research the condition, but rather to minimize alcohol consumption. This is particularly true for the U.S.

In colonial times, the states imposed fines for drunken behavior on the citizens, or for selling alcohol to known drunks. However, alcoholic drinks themselves were not frowned on until the end of the 18th century, when the temperance movement began in earnest. The temperance movement, led by religious leaders like Cotton Mather and John Wesley, first preached against the evils of "fardent spirits," or hard liquor. But leaders like the Irish priest Theobald Matthew and groups like the American Temperance Society started advocating complete abstinence from alcohol by the early 19th century. There was a clear conflict at the end of the Civil War in 1865 between "drys," which advocated the prohibition of alcoholic beverages, and "wets," which did not. Groups like the Woman's Christian Temperance Union, founded in 1874, and the American Anti-Saloon League, founded in 1895, were steadily gaining in political influence. By 1913 nine states had instituted a complete ban on alcohol and many other states had severely restricted the availability of alcohol.

Finally, temperance groups persuaded Congress in 1917 to pass national prohibition. In 1919 the states ratified the 18th Amendment, and on January 27, 1920, the National Prohibition Act, also known as the Volstead Act, came into force. The prohibition lasted for thirteen years, during which time alcoholic beverages were illegally produced, marketed, exported, or smuggled into America.

Prohibition, sometimes called "the experiment of the nobles," was a failure. It forced him underground into illegal speakeasies, rather than eliminating alcohol consumption; by the late 1920s, there were more speakeasies than there had been saloons. Bootlegging liquor became a lucrative, gangster-controlled activity that bribed local police and public officials. Violence and corruption have soared, while the alcohol abuse problem has only got worse. Until 5th December 1933, as the 21st Amendment was passed, the ban was officially repealed.

The attempt by the government to solve alcohol problems alone had failed by law. But the problems remained, and other types of strategies for dealing with alcoholism were developed after the repeal of prohibition. Alcoholics Anonymous is the most famous of these. Founded in the 1930s, today it continues to strive to teach alcoholics how to overcome their addiction and remain sober. More recently, psychological counseling techniques were developed and organizations formed to help people overcome alcoholism, in addition to AA. Further more, there has been a substantial progress in public awareness of the problem; rather than being seen simply as a sinful or irresponsible behavior as it was before prohibition, since the 1930s, more and more people have begun to view alcoholism as a medical problem rather than a vice.

While sympathy for alcoholics has improved, the alcohol problem has not gone away and the opinions of the Americans on alcoholic beverages remain mixed. Following the repeal of prohibition, most states maintained laws that limited the availability of alcohol. Many of these regulations have been expanded in the 1970s: alcoholic beverage taxes have been raised and the legal drinking age has been increased to 21. Some people believed America was entering an era of "neo-prohibitionism" — a public policy shift back to ideals of temperance. Instead, in the mid-1990s, widespread media coverage of the potential health benefits of moderate drinking prompted many to theorize that views had once again changed and that the US was beginning a revived "love affair" with alcohol.

Whatever current American attitudes towards alcohol may be, one thing is certain: millions of them continue to become alcoholics, while countless more experience alcohol abuse-related devastating problems.

The writers in Alcoholism: Current Controversies address the nature of alcoholism and the severity of alcohol-related issues and what should be done to prevent them in the following chapters: How severe are the drug and alcohol abuse problems? Was Alcoholism an Injury? Which successful is the anonymity of alcoholics? Was Alcohol Industry Responsible for Its Products? How to Avoid Alcohol-related Problems? It is hoped that by exploring the issues surrounding alcoholism and alcohol abuse, the readers will better understand why these problems continue to plague human society despite thousands of years of experience with the effects of alcoholic beverages.

1.1 What is Alcoholism?

The most severe form of alcohol abuse is alcoholism and involves drinking habits being unable to manage them. Alcohol use disorder is also commonly referred to as a disorder. The disorder of alcohol use is classified into three categories: mild, moderate, and extreme. Every group has different symptoms and can cause harmful side effects. If left untreated, alcohol abuse of any sort can spiral out of control. Individuals who struggle with alcoholism sometimes feel like they cannot usually work without alcohol. This can lead to a wide range of issues, professional goals, personal issues, relationships and overall health impacts. The serious side effects of chronic alcohol abuse will intensify over time and cause devastating complications.

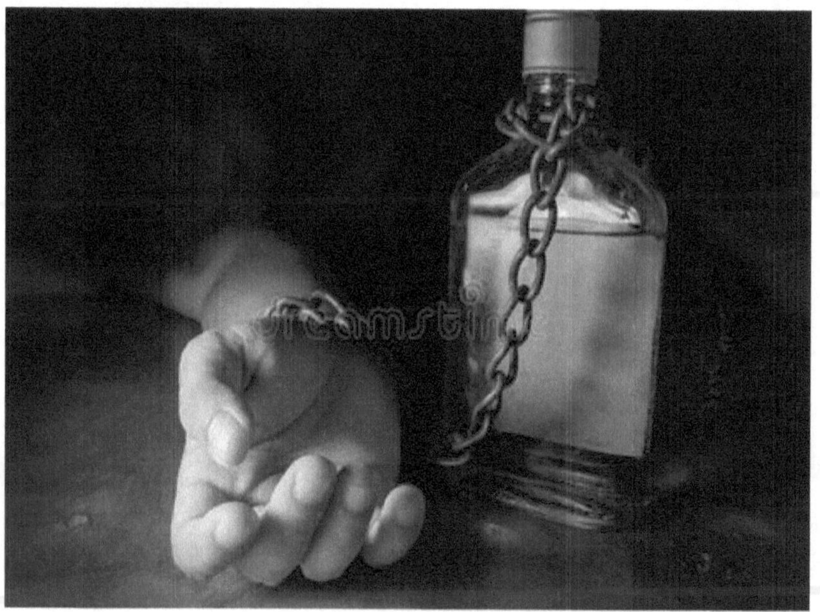

You don't need to be secretly suffering from alcohol addiction. There are a plethora of treatment options readily available to help you overcome alcohol abuse and maintain sobriety over the long term.

1.2 Loss of control

Alcoholism may grow insidiously; there is often no clear line between alcoholism and problem-drinking. The only early signs of alcoholism may be the painful physical withdrawal reactions that occur during even short periods of abstinence. Often people experience long-term depression or anxiety, insomnia, chronic pain, or personal or work-related stress that contributes to alcohol use for relaxation, but often there have been no extraordinary events to reckon for the drinking problem.

Alcoholics usually have little or no control over the amount they are consuming or the length or frequency of drinking. We complain about alcohol, deny their own addiction, and continue to drink even though we know the dangers. With time, some people are unaware of the drinking effects and need more alcohol to become intoxicated, creating the illusion that they can "keep their liquor." While drinking, they experience blackouts and regular hangovers that make them miss work and other normal activities. Alcoholics can drink alone, and begin early in the day.

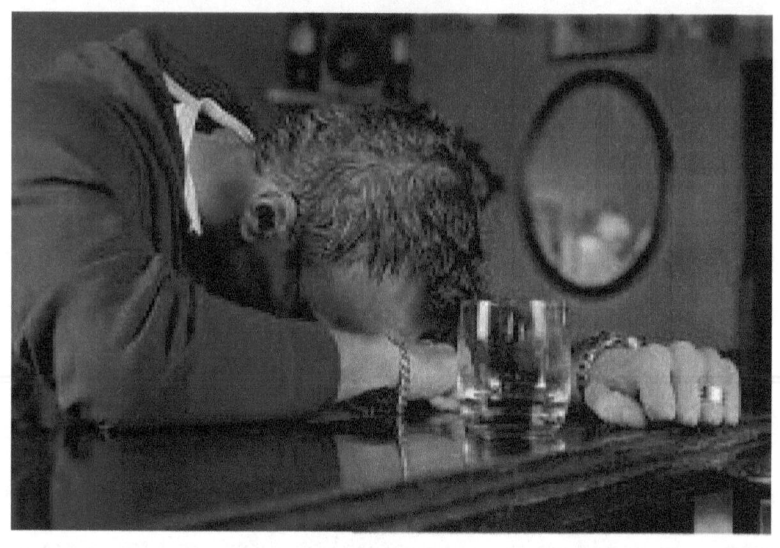

We quit drinking daily or turn from hard liquor to beer or wine, but those times never last.

Severe alcoholics often have a history of injuries, marital and work-related depression and health problems associated with alcohol. Signs of drug or alcohol abuse are often episodic violent and abusive incidents involving spouses and children, and a history of unexplained or recurrent injuries.

Which Alcoholism Causes?

Men have drunk alcohol for 15,000 years. Only drinking regularly and frequently over time may give rise to a sense of dependency and withdrawal symptoms during abstinence periods; however, this physical dependence is not the sole cause of alcoholism. Many factors, including biology and genetics, community, and psychology, typically come into play for developing alcoholism.

1.3 Reasons Why People Drink

There are several factors which can increase the risk of alcohol abuse.

For one cause, people can turn to alcohol, and eventually, develop a drinking dependence.

Drinking during stressful times, for example, — a family death or work loss — can potentially cause long-term substance abuse.

Although there are different reasons why people start drinking, some of the most common are to:

Alleviate stress

Relating to alcohol can affect the probability of developing alcoholism by reducing pressures in everyday life. Since alcohol is both depressive and sedative, drinking gives rise to feelings of pleasure. Frequent drinking, however, creates tolerance which allows you to consume more alcohol to achieve the same effects.

Feel good

Consuming alcohol can provide a break from reality for some people. It provides a sense of relief from the underlying problems that might be trying to escape your mind. Continuous alcohol use, however, can turn into a severe drinking addiction to get through the day or week.

Coping with loss

Losing a family member or friend can emotionally, physically and mentally take a toll on you. Alcohol will relieve sadness and is used to going through difficult times. Depending on the drug, it can turn into a drinking problem, even temporarily.

Many people are simply unable to conquer fear, leading them to worry forever. Drinking reduces the inhibitions of a person and makes them more relaxed in social situations. Nevertheless, this can lead to addictive habits over time.

Lack of Connection

A lot of people drink because they don't feel properly associated with others. They conclude that alcohol will either fill the void or perhaps make forming new bonds easier for them. Yet usually the reverse ends up being accurate.

Shame

Shame is one of the toughest feelings for anyone to deal with, and one of the most painful, too. While alcohol can temporarily cover shame with false emotions, it also causes many individuals to indulge in risky or foolish actions that will later make them feel much more ashamed, which can lead to a spiralling downward.

Trauma

Experts with the treatment of alcoholism experience some form of trauma in nearly every patient they treat. There are many types of trauma, but they all involve traumatic experiences where there was no empathetic witness for the survivor. For many the secret to their healing is the treatment of unresolved trauma.

1.4 The chemistry of the brain and genetic factors

During abstinence, the cravings for alcohol, the pain of withdrawal and the high rate of relapse are due to the brain's tolerance to and reliance on changes in its own chemistry triggered by long-term alcohol use. Alcohol causes relaxation and euphoria but acts on the central nervous system as a depressant too. Even after years of research, scientists do not yet know exactly how alcohol affects the brain or how alcohol affects the brain. Alcohol tends to have major effects on the hippocampus, a brain area associated with learning and memory, and emotion, sensory perception, appetite, and stress control. Alcohol breaks down into compounds that tend to suppress essential neurotransmitters (chemical messengers in the brain) in the hippocampus, called fatty acid ethyl esters. The neurotransmitters gamma-aminobutyric acid (GABA), dopamine, and serotonin are particularly important to alcoholism researchers and are strongly associated with emotional activity and cravings. Research indicates that, in particular, dopamine production is strongly linked to the reinforcing effects of alcohol, nicotine, opiates, and cocaine. Researchers have concentrated on structures of the nerve cells known as Dopamine D2 receptors (DRD2), which influence dopamine production. Mice with few of these receptors have low interest in alcohol and even resistance to it.

Researchers have located a gene in people with severe alcoholism, which alters the role of DRD2. This gene is also found in people at increased risk of alcoholism, and in people with the condition and autism of Tourette. Yet one major study found no link between the DRD2 gene and alcoholism at all. Further work is needed in that field. Researchers are also studying genes that control other enzymes known as kinases that affect the absorption of alcohol in the brain and genes that affect serotonin. Nevertheless, even if genetic factors can be identified, they are unable to account for all cases of alcoholism. Lack of genetic security can potentially play a role in alcoholism. Since alcohol is not readily found in nature, genetic mechanisms to defend against excessive consumption may not have developed in humans, as they often have environmental hazards to protect against.

1.5 Risk factors for alcoholism

Who is an Alcoholic?

General Age and Risks.

Several population studies suggest that between 7.4 percent and 9.7 percent of the population rely on alcohol within a single year, and between 13.7 percent and 23.5 percent of Americans depend on alcohol at some point in their lives. A 1996 national survey found that almost 11 million Americans were heavy drinkers (five or more drinks per time five days a month or more) and 32 million binge drinkers (five or more drinks on one occasion) in the month prior to the study. Individuals with a family history of alcoholism are more likely to start drinking and become intoxicated by age 20. But anyone who starts to drink in puberty runs a higher risk. 1.9 million young people aged 12 to 20 are currently considered heavy drinkers and 4.4 million are binge drinkers. While alcoholism typically occurs in early adulthood, there is no exception for older people. In fact, 15 percent of men and 12 percent of women over 60 drank more than the national standard for excess alcohol intake in one survey. Alcohol also has a different effect on the older body; people who continue the same drinking habits as they age will easily develop a dependency on alcohol without knowing it. While examining the elderly patients, doctors may ignore alcoholism, falsely attributing the symptoms of alcohol abuse to the natural effects of aging.

Sex. Gender.

Many alcoholics are men, but over the past 30 years, the prevalence of alcoholism among women has increased. About 9.5% of men and 2% of women are heavy drinkers, and 22.8% of men are binge drinkers, compared to 8.7% of women. Generally speaking, young women problem drinkers follow their partners ' drinking habits while they appear to indulge in heavy drinking during the premenstrual period. Women tend to become alcoholics later in life than men, and 1.8 million older women are estimated to suffer from alcohol addiction. While heavy drinking usually occurs in women later in life, women's medical problems arise due to the condition. Same age as men, suggesting women are more vulnerable to physical alcohol toxicity.

For sons of intoxicated mothers, the risk of alcoholism is 25%. In women, the family relation is weaker, but genetic factors in both genders lead to this disease. People with alcoholism had appeared to have drinking parents in one study. Women who came from households with a history of emotional disorders, avoiding parents, or upsetting early childhood had no higher risk of drinking than people without such backgrounds. For people at genetic risk, a stable family and psychological health were not safe. Unfortunately, there is no way to determine which intoxicated family members are at the greatest risk of alcoholism.

Irish and Native Americans are at severe risk of alcoholism; American Jews and Asians are at a lower risk. Overall, there is no disparity in the prevalence of alcohol among African Americans, whites and Hispanics. Although the biological causes of such different risks are not transparent, due to the way they metabolize alcohol, certain people in these population groups may be at a greater or lower risk. For example, one Native American study found that they are less responsive to alcohol's intoxicating effects. It contradicts other studies that showed fewer signs of drunkenness in young men with alcoholic fathers and had lower levels of stress hormones than those without a family history. In other words, they'd better "keep their liquor." Experts suggest that such individuals may inherit a lack of those warning signals that usually cause people to stop drinking. On the other hand, many Asians are less likely to become alcoholic due to a genetic factor that makes them deficient in aldehyde dehydrogenase, a chemical which the body uses to metabolize ethyl alcohol.

Upon drinking alcohol, toxic substances build up in its absence and quickly lead to flushing, dizziness and nausea. Therefore, people with this genetic susceptibility are likely to experience adverse alcohol reactions, and thus not become intoxicated. Nevertheless, this deficiency is not entirely protective against drinking, particularly if social pressure is applied, for example among members of the college fraternity. It's important to understand that people with alcoholism are still legally responsible for their actions, whether it is hereditary or not.

Emotional problems.

People with severe depression or anxiety are at high risk for alcoholism, smoking and other types of addictions. Yes, major depression affects nearly one-third of all drug incidents. It is more common among women (and women in general) than men in alcoholics.

Ironically, one study showed depression in alcoholic women can cause them to drink less than non-depressed alcoholic women, whereas depression has the opposite effect in alcoholic people.

Depression and anxiety may play a pivotal role in the development of elderly alcoholism, which is often subject to drastic changes in life, such as retirement, the loss of a spouse or friends, and medical issues. In these cases problem drinking may be due to anxiety or depression self-medication. Nevertheless, it should be remembered that these mood disturbances can in fact be caused by alcoholism in all people with alcoholism and often abate after alcohol withdrawal.

The Traits of Personality.

Studies find that alcoholism is strongly associated with impulsive, excitable, and novelty-seeking behavior and such habits are developed early, if not inherited. Individuals with attention deficit hyperactivity disorder, a disease that includes certain habits, have an increased risk of alcoholism. Children who later become alcoholics or misuse drugs are more likely to be less afraid of new circumstances than others, even if the risk of harm is small. Alcoholics (mostly women) did not show any deficiencies in their reasoning in a mental processing examination but were less able to suppress their responses than non-alcoholics. A family history of passivity and irregular attachment needs was once thought to increase the risk of alcoholism, but studies have not borne the hypothesis out.

Factors of the Socioeconomics. Alcoholism has long been thought to be more common in people with lower levels of education, and in those who were unemployed. Nevertheless, a thorough study carried out in 1996 found that the prevalence of alcoholism among adult welfare recipients was 4.3% to 8.2%, which was equivalent to the 7.4% observed in the general population. There was no difference in prevalence among poor African Americans and poor whites as well. People in low-income groups displayed certain patterns that varied from those of the general population. For example, the heavy drinkers were as many women as men. Excessive drinking in lower income groups may be more dangerous; one study found that it was a major factor in higher death rates among people, especially men, in lower socioeconomic groups compared to higher-group ones.

1.6 How serious is alcoholism

Approximately 100,000 deaths can be traced to drinking in whole or in part a year, and intoxication decreases the life expectancy by 10 to 12 years. Apart from smoking, it's America's most common preventable cause of death. While studies indicate that adults who drink moderately (about one drink a day) have lower mortality rates than their non-drinking peers, with heavy drinking their risk of premature death increases. The security that comes with a moderate intake of alcohol seems to be limited to people over 60 who are at risk for heart disease.

The sooner a person starts drinking heavily, the greater the chance they will develop serious illnesses. Alcoholism can lead to deaths of many people in many different ways, and people who drink excessively have a higher death rate from disease, abuse and some cancers in general. Overexposure. Overdose of the alcohol will lead to death. This is a particular danger to teens who may want to impress their friends with their ability to drink alcohol but are still unable to gage their results.

Accidents, Murder and Suicide. Alcohol plays an important role in over half of all deaths in cars. Less than two drinks will hamper driving ability.

In fact, alcohol increases the risk of accidental injury from many other causes.

Another analysis of patients with an emergency room found that having more than another drink doubled the risk of injury, and more than four drinks increased the risk once. Another study reported that 47 percent of patients treated for accidents were positive for alcohol and 35 percent were intoxicated in emergency room conditions. 75 per cent of those who were intoxicated showed evidence of chronic alcoholism. The condition is the main diagnosis in one quarter of all people who commit suicide, and 67 per cent of all murders include alcohol.

Domestic violence and family side effects. Alcohol abuse is a common result of domestic violence. Research suggests that for women, a history of alcohol abuse in her male partner may be the most serious risk factor for injury from domestic violence. Parental alcoholism also increases the risk of violence and violent behavior towards their children. Children of alcoholics appear to do worse than others academically, have a higher incidence of depression, anxiety, and stress, and a lower self-esteem than peers.

One study found that children between the ages of six and 12 who had been diagnosed with major depression were more likely to have alcoholic parents or relatives than children who were not depressed. Alcoholic families are less cohesive, have more disputes and their members are less confident and articulate than non-alcoholic or alcoholic parents recovering households. In addition to their own inherited likelihood of eventual dependence, one study found that 41 per cent of intoxicated children had serious problems with coping that can be life-long. Adult children are at increased risk for divorce and psychological problems from alcoholic parents. One study concluded that sexual and physical violence are the only incidents with greater psychological impact on the children.

Medical Problems

Alcohol can affect the body in a plethora of ways that it is impossible for the researchers to determine exactly what the drinking effects are. Nevertheless, it is well known that chronic consumption contributes to many, some lethal, problems.

Cardiac disease. Large doses of alcohol can cause irregular heartbeats and even in people without a history of heart disease can increase blood pressure. A major study found those who drank more than three alcoholic drinks a day had higher blood pressure compared to teetotalers. The more alcohol one drinks, the greater the blood pressure rises. Those who had been binge drinkers had the highest blood pressure. A study found that binge drinkers (people who take nine or more drinks once or twice a week) had a two-and - a-half-fold chance of a medical emergency compared with nondrinkers. Chronic alcohol abuse can also harm the heart muscle, leading to cardiac insufficiency; women are particularly vulnerable to this. A recent study indicated that moderate to heavy drinking (more than two bottles of beer or two glasses of wine a day) was a greater risk factor for coronary artery disease than smoking, contrary to many previous reports. Light-drinking (two to six drinks a week) was safe, as in other research. This new study needs more research to confirm or refute. In any case, moderate drinking doesn't seem to give any heart benefit to people who are at low risk for beginning with heart disease.

Cancer.

Causes cancer. Alcohol may not cause cancer but the carcinogenic effects of other substances, such as cigarette smoke, are likely increased. Daily drinking increases the risk of cancer of the lung, esophageal, stomach, pancreatic, colorectal, urinary, liver, and brain, lymphoma, and leukemia. Approximately 75 per cent of esophageal cancers and 50 per cent of mouth, throat and larynx cancers are due to alcoholism. (Wine tends to present less risk to such cancers than alcohol or hard liquor.) Smoking combined with smoking significantly increases the risk of most of these cancers. When women eat as little as one drink a day, they will increase their breast cancer chances by as much as 30%.

Hepatic conditions. The liver is especially vulnerable to alcoholism. About 10-35% of heavy drinkers develop alcoholic hepatitis, and 10-20% develop cirrhosis. Alcohol in the liver transforms to an even more toxic substance, acetaldehyde, which can cause considerable damage. Not eating a variety of alcoholic beverages while drinking and consuming are also factors that increase the risk of liver damage. Persons with alcoholism also have a higher risk of developing hepatitis B and C, possibly chronic liver diseases than can lead to cirrhosis and hepatic cancer...

Mental and cognitive dysfunctions.

Alcohol has significant effects on the brain. One research scanning the brains of inebriated subjects revealed that while alcohol activates certain reward-related parts of the brain and causes euphoria, it does not seem to impair cognitive ability (capacity to think and reason). Nevertheless, chronic drug use ultimately causes depression and frustration. Gray matter is lost in chronic situations, contributing probably to insanity and mental disorders. Alcohol can also cause milder neurological problems including headache and insomnia (especially after drinking red wine). Neurological damage is not permanent except in severe cases and abstinence almost always leads to a return of normal mental function. Alcohol can increase the risk of hemorrhagic stroke (caused by bleeding in the brain), though it can protect against stroke from narrowed arteries....

Wernicke-Korsakoff Syndrome and Malnutrition. A pint of whiskey contains about half the daily calories an adult requires, but it has no nutritional value. Alcohol can also interfere with the absorption of proteins, vitamins and other nutrients, in addition to replacing food. A significant deficiency of B-vitamin thiamine, which can cause a serious condition called the WernickeKorsakoff syndrome, is of particular concern in alcoholism. Symptoms of this condition include extreme loss of balance, memory loss and uncertainty. Eventually it can lead to permanent brain damage and death. Another significant nutritional issue among alcoholics is the B vitamin folic acid deficiency which can cause severe anemia....

Interactions of Drugs. Alcohol increases the effectiveness of many drugs, thus inhibiting others. The calming effect on antianxiety narcotics, sedatives, antidepressants, and antipsychotic drugs is of particular importance.

Alcohol also interacts with a number of the medications that diabetics use. It interferes with drugs that prevent seizures or blood clotting. This increases the risk of gastrointestinal bleeding in people taking aspirin or other inflammatory nonsteroidal drugs, including ibuprofen and naproxene. Or put it another way, taking almost every drug would avoid drinking alcohol.

Infant Growth and Pregnancy. Also small levels of alcohol may have adverse effects on the developing fetus including low birth weight and increased risk of miscarriage. High amounts can cause syndrome of fetal alcohol which can lead to retardation of mental and development. One study shows a significantly higher risk of leukemia in female infants who consume any kind of alcohol during pregnancy.

Among Older People, problems. When people age, it takes fewer drinks to get drunk, and smaller amounts of alcohol will affect the organs than younger ones. Up to half of the 100 most prescribed drugs for older people often adversely respond to alcohol.

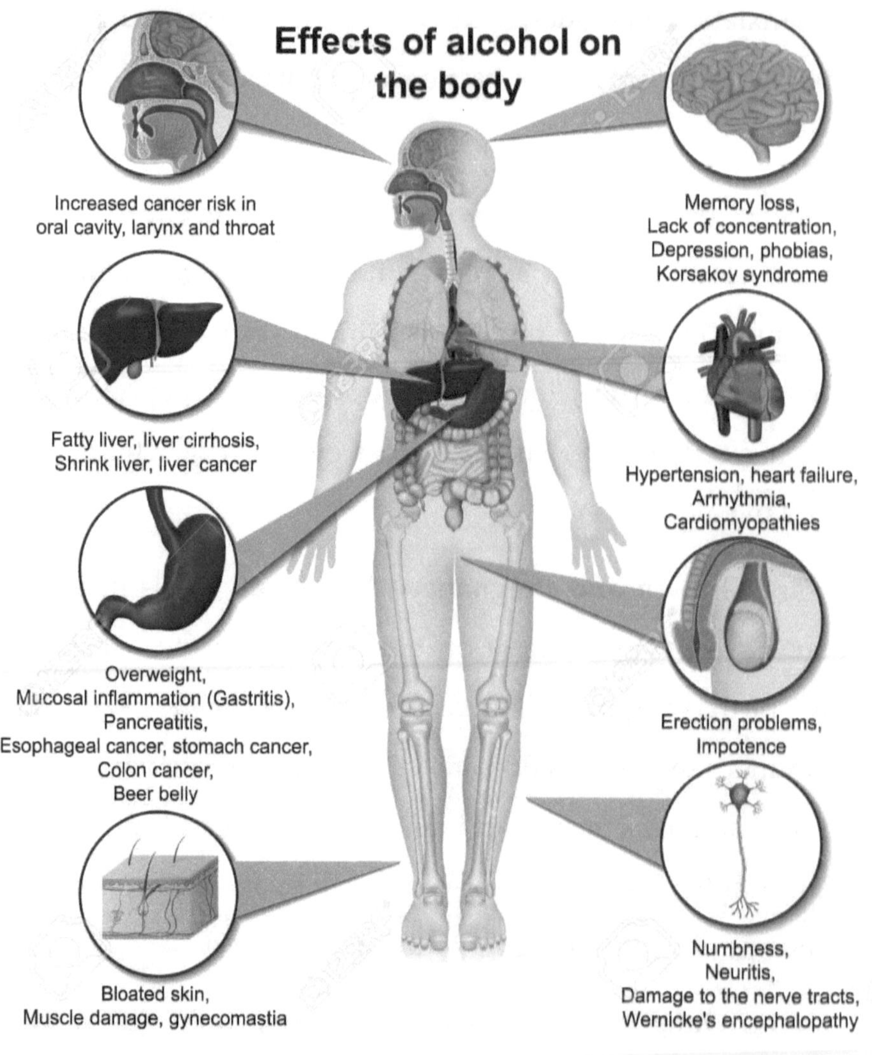

1.7 Getting treatment

Even if people with alcoholism experience symptoms of withdrawal, they almost always deny the problem, leaving it up to family, friends or relatives to identify the symptoms and take the first steps towards recovery....

A study reported that the main reasons alcoholics are not seeking treatment are lack of trust in effective treatments, denial of their own alcoholism and the social stigma attached to the disorder and its treatment. Some studies have found that even a brief intervention (e.g., multiple 15-minute therapy sessions with a doctor and follow-up by a nurse) can be very effective in reducing drinking in non-dependent heavy drinkers. The best methods, however, are group meetings between alcoholics and their friends and family members who have been affected by alcoholic behavior. Using this interventional approach, each affected person gives a caring yet straightforward and frank report explicitly explaining how their loved one or friend's alcoholism directly harmed him or herself. Even children may be involved in this process, depending on their maturity level and ability to handle the situation. The family and friends should communicate their love for the patient and their willingness to help the patient during rehabilitation, but they must insist that the patient seek treatment actively and faithfully. It can be particularly effective for employers. An approach should also be sensitive yet firm, endangering the employee with job loss if he or she is not seeking help. Many large companies give their employees access to cheap or free treatment programs.

The alcoholic patient and all concerned should fully understand that alcoholism is a disease, and that the reactions to this disease — need, cravings, fear of withdrawal — are not character flaws, but symptoms, just as pain or discomfort are symptoms of other conditions. We should also know that recovery is complicated and sometimes unpleasant, just as treatments are for other life-threatening illnesses, such as cancer, but that this is the only chance for a cure.

The withdrawal symptoms.

When a person with alcoholism stops drinking, the symptoms of withdrawal begin within 6 to 48 hours and occur about 24 to 35 hours after the last drink. During this time the alcohol-induced suppression of brain activity is suddenly reversed. Stress hormones are over-produced, and over-excited the central nervous system. Approximately 5 percent of intoxicated patients experience delirium tremens, typically two or four days after the last drink.

Symptoms include fever, rapid heartbeat, high or low blood pressure, extremely aggressive behavior, hallucinations and other mental disorders.

Tremens Recovery, Seizures and Other Severe Symptoms. Individuals with delirium tremens signs should be treated immediately. Untreated delirium tremors have a fatality rate of up to 20%. We are usually given anti-anxiety drugs intravenously for the first time, and their physical condition is stabilized. It is vitally important to administer fluids. It may require vigilance to prevent injury to themselves or others.

1.8 Long term treatment and relapse

The two main long-term counseling goals are total abstinence and substitution of addictive habits with appropriate, time-filling activities that can fill the void in the daily activity that exists after drinking has stopped. Several studies have shown that some people who are dependent on alcohol will eventually learn how to regulate and do their drinking, as well as those who remain abstinent. Nevertheless, there is no way to determine which individuals will quit after one drink and which cannot. Alcoholics Anonymous and other organizations in drug recovery whose aim is absolute abstinence are greatly concerned about the ads surrounding these findings, as many individuals with alcoholism are looking for an excuse to start drinking. At this time the only safe route is abstinence....

Why Do People Relapse From Alcoholism?

Even after years of abstinence, between 80 percent and 90 percent of people treated for alcoholism recur. Patients and their families should understand that alcoholism relapses are similar to frequent flare-ups with chronic physical illnesses. One study found that there were three factors that put a person at high risk of relapse: frustration and anger, social pressure and internal temptation. Nevertheless, treatment of relapses doesn't always require detoxification or hospitalization starting from scratch; abstinence can often start the next day. Self-sufficiency and resilience are essential habits for permanent recuperation.

Emotional and mental pain. Alcohol prevents emotional pain and is often viewed as a loyal friend in the absence of human relations. It is also related to independence and a lack of inhibition that reduces the tedium of daily routines.

When the addict decides to quit drinking, the brain seeks to regain what it sees as its equilibrium. Depression and anxiety (the mental correlates of physical pain) are the best brain tools toward abstinence that tend to encourage alcoholics to return to drinking even after signs of physical withdrawal have abated. In this phase, only intellect is no help, for the brain will use all its rationalizing forces to convince the individual to return to drinking. It's important to realize that any change in life will cause temporary sadness and anxiety, even for the better. This emotional turmoil weakens over time and the replacement of healthy pleasures and can be resolved.

One of the most challenging problems a person with alcoholism faces is being around people who can drink socially without the danger of being addicted. A sense of alienation, a lack of pleasure, and the perception of the ex-drinker that pity— not respect — is driving the disposition of a friend that can lead to depression, low self-esteem, and a strong desire to drink. Close friends and even intimate partners may find it difficult to change their attitudes to this newly sober person and, worse, still may promote a return to alcohol. To maintain alcoholic relationships, partners frequently develop their self-images on maintaining or managing the questionable actions of their mates and then find that abstinence threatens them.

Colleagues may not readily accept the sober, perhaps more reserved, comrade. In such situations, survival can require separation from these "enablers." It's no wonder a person returns to alcohol when faced with such losses, even if they are temporary.

In these situations, the best course is to urge close friends and family members to seek help too. Fortunately, for this reason, programs such as Al-Anon exist.

From social and cultural industries. Through advertisements and programming, the media depicts the benefits of alcohol. The medical advantages of light to moderate drinking are widely advertised, which offers ex-drinkers the bogus justification for their wellbeing to resort to alcohol. Such advertisements have to be categorically dismissed and known for what they are— the effort by an organization to benefit from the tremendous potential damage to individuals.

Chapter 2: The Sufferings Of Children Of Alcoholics And Alcoholic Teenagers

One in five adult Americans had grown up living with an alcoholic. Child and adolescent psychologists realize these children are at greater risk than children whose parents are not alcoholics for having emotional issues. Alcoholism runs in families, and alcoholic children are four times more likely to become alcoholics than other children. Many addicted children have endured some form of neglect or abuse.

A kid in a family like that can have a number of problems: • Guilt. The child may perceive itself or herself as the main cause of drinking from the mother or father.

Angst. The child can constantly worry about the domestic situation. He or she may fear that the intoxicated parent will become sick or injured, and may also fear fights and parental abuse.

Confusion. Parents can give the child the impression that an awful secret is present at home. The embarrassed child does not invite friends over and avoids asking for help from anyone.

Inability to maintain close relations. Because the drinking parent has disappointed the child several times, he or she is also distrustful of others.

Merger. The intoxicated parent will suddenly change from caring to furious, no matter the actions of the child. There is no regular daily routine, which is very important for a child, since bedtime and mealtimes change constantly.

Hot. The child is angry with the alcoholic parent for drinking and maybe upset with the non-alcoholic parent for lack of protection and care.

Tumbling. The child feels alone and unable to turn the situation around.

2.1. Warning Signs

Although the child tries to keep a secret about alcoholism, teachers, family, other adults or peers can know something is wrong. Child and adolescent therapists warn that the following activities can indicate a drinking or other problems at home: • School failure; truancy

- Lack of friends; isolation from classmates

- Delinquent behavior, such as theft or assault

- Physical symptoms, like headaches or stomach aches

- Drug abuse or alcohol abuse

- Aggression against other children

- Risk-taking behaviors

By becoming managed, successful "overachievers" throughout the school, they can cope with alcoholism while being emotionally disconnected from other children and teachers at the same time. Their emotional problems can only manifest when they become adults.

Whether or not their parents seek alcohol treatment, these children and adolescents may benefit from educational programs and organizations of mutual assistance such as alcoholic children's programs, Al-Anon, and Alateen.

Prompt, professional help is also critical in preventing the child from having more serious problems, including alcoholism. Child and adolescent psychiatrists support these children with their own issues and also help the child realize that they are not responsible for their parents' drinking problems.

The treatment therapy may include group therapy with other youths, minimizing alienation from being an addicted teen. The child and adolescent therapist will often work with the whole family to help them establish healthier ways to relate to each other, particularly when the intoxicated parent has stopped drinking.

2.2. Alcohol – most common gateway for teenagers

Alcohol is considered as the most commonly used and abused substance by young people. Marijuana kills more adolescents than all other drugs combined, and is a factor among 15–24 year-olds in the three leading causes of death: injuries, murders and suicides. Nearly four million teenagers suffer from alcohol dependence, which accounts for more than one-fifth of all alcohol-dependent people.

Alcohol can cause severe and life-threatening complications for children and adolescents and can be a precursor to other use of drugs.

The average age children start drinking today is around 13 years old.

The number of 8th, 10th and 12th graders who report having had a drink in the past 30 days, or who have been intoxicated in the past two weeks, has steadily risen since hitting a low point in the early 1990s. Alcohol is the "gateway" drug most widely used by children and teenagers. The word "gateway drug" refers to medications that are the first to be used in a use continuum whose use is correlated statistically with the use of other drugs. If the use of these first drugs can be avoided or postponed until the end of puberty, the probability that people will continue to use other drugs will be greatly reduced, according to the definition of "gateway drugs."

Public health experts have discussed for decades whether there is a link between children's intake of beer, wine coolers and other drinks, smoking cigarettes, and the resulting use of other substances such as marijuana, cocaine, and heroin. In 1994, former Health, Education and Welfare Secretary Joseph A. Califano, Jr., and his organization the Center on Addiction and Substance Abuse at Columbia University (CASA) conducted a systematic nationwide study of the relationship of these gateway drugs to subsequent substance use.

The study showed a powerful statistical link the, in Califano's words, is "far more powerful than[the statistical connections] that first exposed the correlation between smoking and lung cancer and emphysema, between cholesterol levels and heart disease, and between exposure to asbestos and lung cancer." Although everyone who drinks won't progress to other drugs, everyone who uses "has a strong connection"

In its report, CASA found even more disturbing evidence: more than 67 percent of people who start drinking before the age of fifteen ends up using an illicit drug, while less than 25 percent of those who avoid drinking until the age of seventeen or older advance to other substances. Of those who never drink, just 4% end up using other drugs.

Children aged 12 to 17 who drink are 22.3 times more likely than those who don't drink to smoke marijuana, and they are 50 times more likely to use cocaine.

To parents, to mayors and city councils, and for federal drug prevention efforts, the message is very clear: if children avoid drinking until it's legal to do so, they're almost certain to make it through life without using illicit drugs.

2.3. Trends of early age drinking

It is no surprise that children and youngsters are consuming alcoholic beverages, just how much they are drinking and how often a discovery can be. Three out of five teenagers across the nation have had a drink in the last month (61 per cent). Boys under the age of 17 drink more heavily than any other population group: nearly three out of ten (29 per cent) drink six or more alcoholic beverages each time they drink, compared with 24 per cent of 18 and 19 year-olds.

The 1998 "Monitoring the Future Study," a national survey funded by the National Institute of Drug Abuse and carried out by the Institute of Social Research, reveals that 8th, 10th and 12th graders are all far more likely to have used alcohol in the past 30 days or the past year than they are to have smoked marijuana or used any other illicit drug. In 1998, alcohol was experimented by 44 per cent of 8th graders, 63 per cent of 10th graders and 74 per cent of 12th graders. This compares with 17% of 8th graders, 31% of 10th graders and 38% of 12th graders who have experimented with marijuana.

Most teens drink: a recent survey of 4,390 seniors and dropouts from high school found that approximately 80 percent reported drinking, binge drinking, or drinking and driving in the previous year.

Alcohol is available readily. Alcohol is the most easily obtainable drug for children. 25-30 per cent of 6th graders said in a recent student study in Washington State that it would be easy for them to get a beer, wine or hard liquor. This compares with around 6-7 percent who say it's easy to get marijuana and 0 percent who report it's easy to get cocaine, LSD or amphetamines. As children grow older, they generally find it easier to find drugs, but alcohol remains the most accessible: 55% of 8th graders say alcohol is easy to obtain compared to 25-39% who could easily find marijuana and 10-15% who could easily find other drugs. More than one in five seniors in high school (22 percent) report a recent heavy alcohol use compared to one in seven (15 percent) who report recent heavy marijuana use.

Beer is considered as the alcoholic drink of choice for children, preferred by 61 per cent of all kids. 27 percent of all children prefer the next favorite alcoholic-beverage, wine and wine coolers. In 1991 the United States Inspector General The Department of Health and Human Services reported that every year junior and senior high school students drank 1.1 billion cans of beer and 300 million bottles of wine-coolers.

Drinking binge. Most adults imagine drinking after work as a leisurely cocktail or beer, or an elegant glass of wine with dinner. Unfortunately, that's not the way children drink. People are much more likely to "drink to get drunk" as people drink. According to a 1995 Harvard School of Public Health College Drug Survey, 52 percent of college students were "binge drink" up from 33 per cent in 1993. According to a report by the American Academy of Pediatrics, the amount of drinking and the amounts consumed are superb: the average teen drinks on more than five days a month. Kids who drink also consume an average of 5.6 drinks at a time. Binge drinking starts early: 39 per cent of seniors in high school report having at least once in the previous month five or more drinks at a time.

Binge drinking is a major health issue— and in the past year has led to a number of widely publicized deaths among college students. It is also important in the role of alcohol as a gateway to other drugs: the more alcohol a child consumes, the greater the likelihood that they will turn toward other drugs.

2.4. Consequences of early age drinking

While drinking at any age poses health risks, certain risks are specific to minors. A 1997 study carried by researchers at the National Institute on Alcohol Abuse and Alcoholism (NIAAA) found that the age one begins drinking has a dramatic impact on the chances of developing alcohol dependence. People taking their first drink at age 13 have a 47.3 percent chance of becoming dependent on alcohol over their lifetime. The chances drop to 30.6 percent for those who postpone drinking until age 16; those who wait until age 21 have only a 10.0 percent chance of developing alcohol dependence.

The sooner one drinks, the more likely it is that other substances will end up using. Research suggests that the majority of those starting to drink between 13 and 16 would move toward other drugs.

Young brains are more susceptible to damage from the alcohol than fully mature brains. Within adolescent brains, alcohol shrinks memory signals much faster (at a lower dose) than in the adult brain, and decreases memory development. Those who are exposed to alcohol in puberty display a decreased ability to learn as opposed to those who are exposed to adult alcohol.

Alcohol consumption has been shown in animal studies to delay the onset of puberty, resulting in sluggish bone growth, and weaker bones.

Fatalities in traffic. Among 15 to 20-year-olds, motor vehicle crashes are the leading cause of death. In 1997, 3,336 drivers died between the ages of 15 and 20, in motor vehicle accidents about 365,000 were injured. About 30 per cent of those drivers were intoxicated. The economic cost calculated for those accidents was $31.9 billion.

Younger drivers are more likely than older drivers to have been binge drinking (39% vs. 13%) and are more likely to have had both their first and last drinks in less than an hour (30% vs. 15%).

Both states and the Columbia district now have minimum drinking age requirements of 21 years old. The National Highway Traffic Safety Administration states that these regulations have decreased traffic fatalities among drivers aged 18 to 20 by 13 per cent and since 1975 have saved an additional 17,359 lives.

Suicide and alcohol: Suicide is now the second-largest cause of death in the United States for children aged 15 to 19.

Adolescent use of alcohol has been related to contemplating, preparing, attempting and achieving suicide. The more often an adolescent consumes alcohol, the greater the likelihood they will contemplate or attempt suicide; alcohol is more closely correlated with suicidal thoughts than any other substance, and more closely linked to actual attempts at adolescent suicide than any other drug other than crack cocaine. For one survey, 37 percent of females in the 8th grade who drank heavily reported attempting suicide, compared to 11 percent who did not drink

2.5. Alcohol consumptions result in social problems

Problems of Drugs and Health. Drinking leads to school troubles.

High school youth who are regular users of drugs are three to five times more likely than non-users to have given up on school, to have dropped out of school at some point, to have been suspended in the last year, and to find good grades unimportant. Regular users often participate less in athletics or other extracurricular activities.

In 40 percent of academic problems, 28 percent of dropouts and 80 percent of acts of vandalism, drug use by college students is a factor. Alcohol is associated with 95 per cent of violent crime on college campuses. 90 per cent of all campus rapes reported involve alcohol use by the victim or perpetrator.

Alcohol and Juvenile Abuse. Alcohol and violence go hand in hand too. Many offenders sentenced to prison have a history of substance abuse; alcohol is the most widely used drug. Of 1,030 teenagers aged 12 to 17 who joined the services of the Texas Youth Commission, alcohol was the most common drug used. The following table offers a summary of substance use in the year prior to the month before entering the facility: alcohol 26.9% Cannabis 22.5% Cocaine (powder) 15.6% Inhalants 12.5% Downers 10.4% Uppers 9.3% Crack 6.4% Heroin 4.2% Most assume that the drug most used by juvenile offenders is crack cocaine.

The National Institute of Justice's 1997 Annual Report on Adult and Juvenile Arrestees tells a different story. The average age at which offenders first began using alcohol ranged from 14.1 (Houston) to 15.8 (Miami— results are reported to be city by city), while the average age at which offenders started using crack ranged from 23.3 (Houston) to 28.2 (Atlanta) years. Apparently, alcohol is the drug of choice for juvenile offenders as well as the youth population in general.

Women and alcohol. Alcohol consumption is also more likely to lead to risky sexual behavior: high school students who drink are four times more likely to have had sexual intercourse, and twice as likely as non-drinkers to have four or more partners, habits that increase the risk of sexually transmitted diseases, including HIV.

Drinking caused health problems. Young people suffer the same long-term health risks that older drinkers do: alcohol is the United States' third leading cause of death. Men and women who regularly drink alcoholic beverages have higher death rates from cirrhosis, mouth cancer, larynx, pharynx, oesophagus, and liver compared to abstainers; colorectal cancer, breast cancer, hemorrhagic stroke; and injury, abuse, poisoning, and suicide.

Alcohol causes birth defects and can cause pancreatic inflammation and brain damage. In people at risk of coronary artery disease, the intake of small amounts of alcohol can provide some offsetting health benefits — but generally, young people are not at risk in coronary artery disease.

This perspective focuses on children's use of alcohol, but their parents' use of alcohol is an equally significant issue for children and society at large. CASA estimates that alcohol or other drug abuse and addiction cause or worsen at least seven out of ten cases of child abuse and neglect.

Any comprehensive national program to minimize or avoid alcohol and drug addiction issues must deal with parents' alcohol consumption as well as children's consumption.

2.6. Binge drinking on college campuses

McCray says that the typical way he drinks is his birthday party. But it does reflect the way too many foresee and experience drinking at college. Surveys show that up to 85 percent of all college students are imbibed, and that almost half are heavily intoxicated.

When the first comprehensive study of college drinking was made in 1949, the undergraduates drank their age no more than others, and college life did not encourage unnecessary tipping. It could not be said the same today.

Students at the college drink more because officials at the college are less stringent and many young people drink at or before high school. The consequence is that students are now meeting communities in college where drinking is not only normal but is done primarily to get drunk.

- Tend to react with hand wringing, claiming they can do little.

- Research, including a United States study News & World Report, says it is not. U.S. News received responses from 69 percent of the 1,320 four-year college and university presidents it surveyed to learn what makes a difference. The survey found that while college presidents tend to highlight the dangers of alcohol abuse among students, many don't see how popular binge drinking really is.

- Almost 3% of the presidents answering the questionnaire reported a rate as high as that found by a study at Harvard University and, surprisingly, 21% couldn't tell how popular it was on their campuses. Many experts suggest that teaching students when to say when is a good idea;

others say schools may even better forbid them to drink. The U.S. News study and follow-up reports suggest that schools authorizing on-campus drinking are up to three times more likely to experience high numbers of binge drinkers.

- In college don't just drop more alcohol, experts say; others also swell stronger kinds, including "PGA" (pure grain alcohol) and potent concoctions of several alcoholic beverages — sometimes through funnels or directly from the keg taps, when hanging upside down. "When I was at school if you got drunk once a week, you were assumed to be someone with whom no one wanted to hang out, never mind[getting drunk] three or four times a week," says Fran Cohen, 52, director of the Student Life Office at Rhode Island University.

- She's dealing with students who don't seem to be aware of drunken behavior, wooziness, vomiting, and passing that goes with too much alcohol.

- Late-fall fraternity party at the University of DePauw in Greencastle, Indiana, is proving her point. Guests–many of whom had already buzzed at smaller parties and in the football match against rival Wabash College–hurled empty beer bottles from the Delta Tau Delta house balcony, watching them break in the courtyard. Their goal was the fraternity crest, and when a big bash was going on guests knew how to walk far away from the area. Within, several hundred people, many sitting on the back of another, were shouting over the throbbing bass of the stereo. Men and women were waiting for their turns to lie on their backs and get beer or schnapps poured into their mouths from a whistle, the prize of the football victory that day.

- Or she rose to the cheers of the audience and the clanking of the bell after each student gulped — be it one or 12. In the meantime, a nauseated woman leaning over plastic trash can support her for a couple of minutes, a man holding her so she wouldn't hit her headfirst.

- Scientists call this "binge drinking," which is described as five or more drinks for a man at any time within a span of two weeks, four or more for a woman.

- The term does not mean getting dropped-down drunk, says Dr Henry Wechsler, the principal investigator in the college drinking study at Harvard. Alternatively, consuming five drinks in a row is indicative of drinking problems. However, he found that few students who eat five will struggle to drink six or more. It's right there, it's safe, it's in front of you and the next thing you know you've got 12 drinks in an hour and you can't move about," describes one senior college participant.

- Harvard study found that 44 per cent of all binge drink undergraduates in the U.S. — a rate that has been fairly constant for nearly 20 years. It also showed that 23 per cent of men and 17 per cent of women were regular binge drinkers — downing three or more times every two weeks with a bunch of drinks.

Behavior

- A lot of drinking is taking its toll. Tim Anderl, a senior at Ohio University, usually says, "You're shattered by the end of the fall and your grades are in the gutter." However, many students spend more money on alcohol in a semester— over $300— than they do on books. There is a link between alcohol and grades, as well. Another study found that A students have three drinks a week on average, while those who make D's and F's 11 drinks a week on average.

- Issues aren't the only ones plaguing binge drinkers. They are two to five times as likely to engage in unplanned or unprotected sex, get sick, damage property, dispute, fight, or face police trouble as other drinkers do.

- A few die. Scott Krueger, 18, a highly accomplished student at the Massachusetts Institute of Technology, overdosed in September 1997 at a fraternity party, slipped into a coma and died three days later. Leslie Anne Baltz was an honorary 21-year-old student at the University of Virginia until November when she drank too much at a pregame party, was left alone by friends to sleep it off, somehow fell down a flight of stairs, hit her head, and died. During the fall term 1997, alcohol poisoning or alcohol-related accidents killed at least five other undergraduates nationally.

- Nobody counts the number of college students who die from drug use, George Mason University's Dr David Anderson in Fairfax, Virginia, reports that at least 50 die each year.

- Drinkers also complicate life for students who don't drink too heavily. In schools where over 50% of students binge drink, Wechsler found that most non-bingeing students complain about the second-hand consequences of binge drinking, ranging from "from abuse to sexual assault to theft to just being a pain all around."

- **<u>Alcohol abuse on college campuses</u>**

- Administrators also consider alcohol abuse amongst students as one of their biggest challenges. But, on the rise until 1994, funding for prevention programs never reached more than a few dollars per pupil, not including wages for employees. Researchers argue that many alcohol education services seldom include more than a few posters, several brochures, and Drug Awareness Week, all of which are largely ignored by students.

- DeJong, CEO of the Boston-based Higher Education Center for Alcohol and Other Drug Prevention, thinks that colleges need to improve how they attract students. "We will draw a particular kind of student if their view books show scenes of small groups socializing rather than football games, tailgate parties and so on," he claims. The U.S. News study of college presidents shows that they were around half as likely to have high levels of binge drinkers when colleges included their drug policies and the related sanctions in the recruitment materials.

- The approach the University of Rhode Island is pursuing once a top party school has been ranked. On a bright fall afternoon, URI junior Denis Guay takes a tour of the campus to a freshman dormitory room for prospective students and their parents. After pointing the route to the toilets, he notes the alcohol policy of the school: no drinking by anyone under the age of 21 anywhere on campus and only one six-pack at a time per student of legal age in the dormitories. The first violation receives a $50 fine; the second, $100; and the third, a suspension.

- And Judi Kroll were delighted to hear of the low tolerance alcohol policy on the tour with their son Jon. Jon questioned that the steps had indeed been applied.

- A number of URI students said it was possible to drink discreetly on campus, they shared more with sophomore Kira Edler, who said, "If you get caught, rates are payable." As a consequence, URI is less of a party school. Since 1990 onwards, kegs were banned from campus, alcohol was banned from social events, and fines were imposed and raised. While the number of alcohol possession violations is on the rise, other alcohol-related crimes, such as abuse or vandalism, have dropped sharply. The concern against such legislation has always been that it drives underground drinking. Wechsler, from Harvard, claims that managers who claim they are shunning accountability. "If you let them drink on campus, that doesn't mean that they're just going to drink on campus," he says. He believes that campuses have less binge drinking, as students are allowed to concentrate on other activities. One explanation might be that schools with such strict policies on anti-drinking attract fewer students who want to party.

- Number of students at Earlham College in Richmond, Indiana, said their decision to attend the liberal arts college was motivated by dry policy of the school.

- Thing I like about that is that you can stop it if you don't want to see alcohol," says student Roscoe Klausing.

- More restrictive policies— which are recorded by 30 percent of U.S. campuses. In the last two years, reporting has done — it's no panacea. Consistent compliance is important, as is filling the days and nights with meaningful activities for students. On too many campuses, Friday classes are a joke, and grade inflation has allowed students to spend even less time on the coursework. "Nothing else to do but drink" is a popular lament among students at the college.

- General, presidents of colleges in urban areas, record lower binge drinking rates on campus than those operating schools in less urban settings, where there are more social and cultural opportunities to attract students. Furthermore, schools with lots of older or part-time students record low binge-drinking levels, possibly because the students have families, careers, or commitments that hold them away from the party circuit.

- **<u>Fraternity at colleges</u>**

- Experts agree that abuse of alcohol is perhaps most common and causes the most problems in areas where schools have little or no control, such as the network of fraternities. Studies show that members of the fraternity and sorority row are three to four times as likely as other students to be binge drinkers, and their representatives are among the most likely.

- In order to encourage drinking an organization need not be Greek. At St. John's University, an all-male Catholic college in central Minnesota, the unofficial rugby club at the school introduced its new members one freezing Saturday night at an off-campus party house known as the Far Side by the locals. The behavior is as surreal as a drawing by Gary Larson. A "Drink Chant, [expletive]!" Expletive] Drink! Expletive] Drink! Drink it!" Ringing. Two beer kegs hang out while Jack Daniels waits for the rookies of the squad on a table inside a fifth — boys dressed only in bras and panties. St. John's officials say the event is not common there and they've worked with the rugby team to discuss options for new members to be introduced.

- The activity has often earned little more than a "boys will be boys" response at most schools, however, before student injuries or deaths, as well as litigation and rising insurance premiums, cause some action. Nationally, by 2000, two brotherhoods committed to having dry quarters. In December, all of the National Inter-fraternity Conference's 66 affiliate fraternities passed a resolution proposing chapter houses without alcohol. Carothers from URI have relocated all but two brotherhoods to campus, where they have to comply with the rules of school. The Inter-fraternity Council of the University of Iowa has requested that official Greek parties be alcohol-free starting next fall.

- Some colleges and Greek groups are making headway; they tend to be much less cooperative in the pubs and liquor stores outside colleges. One senior at Cornell University says, "I was 17 when I first went to school and could get a drink anywhere," including several bars and convenience stores near campus, where students sometimes show false proof of age. College newspaper ads lure students with "Nickel Beer," "Beat the Clock," and "Penny' to You Pee" nights where drinks are discounted or served with a small cover charge. Senior Anthony Antonino insisted in the crowded parking lot outside of Caesar's, an ocean-side bar running a busy "Slug Fest" special about 5 miles from URI, that when he had to interrupt himself, the students there knew their drinking limit. "Oh, my divinity!" He screamed out. "Ok, there's an exception." He pointed to a young woman just squatting on a car's front wheel to relieve herself.

Norm needs to be changed

- College administrators have joined community leaders on committees dubbed "town and gown" to deal with this and other problems. Experts say schools will use their economic clout to force intervention by local governments and alcohol control boards. The Higher Education Alliance for Alcohol and Other Drug Prevention president's leadership group goes a step further, encouraging their peers to advocate for more stringent laws at the state level. A peeved Bill Sheen is conscious that such measures are working. The sophomore business major was fined $195 for holding a cup of Soda and Jim Beam whisky outside a rowdy apartment party after the Tallahassee police began their weekend "Party Patrol." "Sucking. We are not permitted to have a band, "he says.

- And universities will never completely rid themselves of alcohol abuse, says Wechsler; rather, the goal is to shift the rule. Look what's happened to smoking. With few complaints, the signs "No Smoking" are obeyed.

- Designated driver, a concept unheard of fifteen years ago, is now a common practice, even for college kids who are drinking. Some of the more moderate drinkers have had drug awareness, experts say. Now it is time to reach for heavy drinkers.

Chapter 3: Is Alcoholism a disease?

Most experts disagree as to whether drinking is an addiction or simply a bad habit. Supporters of the disease model, including the American Medical Association, claim that alcoholics are victims of a medical condition that occurs in individuals with certain hereditary disease risk factors, such as genetic predisposition or irregular brain chemistry. Those who oppose this view believe that alcoholism is not a biological disorder, but rather a self-destructive behavior that can be resolved by a person through willpower and therapeutic advice.

The concept of the disease first gained widespread acceptance after E.M's 1960 publication. Jellinek's book The Theory of Alcoholism in Disease. Jellinek maintained that some alcoholics have a disorder, but not all. Many alcoholics become physically dependent on alcohol and suffer serious health problems as a result of their drinking; Jellinek argued that this type of alcoholism is an unintentional disorder that is detrimental to one's health, and thus a disease. Nevertheless, he was quick to note that some heavy drinkers don't become dependent on alcohol, and others may be dependent on drinking mentally but not physically.

Jellinek postulated that an unknown biological cause had led to the development of the disease state in some drinkers but not others. Most researchers now conclude that this unknown risk factor could be the genetic makeup of a person: "Twin and adoption studies have, with unusual exception, indicated that genetic factors play an important role in alcohol etiology," says physician Kenneth Kendler.

Supporters of the disease model reject the idea that in some people, alcoholism occurs simply because they have a specific biological structure. Actually, they think alcoholics are drinking as a way to deal with other issues in their lives. Alcoholism is, according to this view, a pattern of behavior, one that is also influenced by social and cultural influences. Researcher George E. Valliant, for example, found the Irish were seven times more likely to develop alcoholism in one group of Irish and Italian neighbors. Valliant postulated that this was not due to genetic differences, but rather because "It is consistent with Irish culture to see the use of alcohol in terms of black or white, good or bad, drunkenness or total abstinence, whereas in Italian culture it is the distinction between moderate drinking and intoxication that is most significant."

The authors address the relative importance of these variables in the following sections, and the advantages and disadvantages of the alcoholism disease model.

3.1. Doctors must treat alcoholism as a disease

The controversy about whether alcoholism is a disorder or a question of personal conduct has been going on for more than 200 years. In the United States, in 1784, Benjamin Rush, M.D., was credited with first describing alcoholism as a "disease." He concluded that alcohol was the causative agent, the signature symptom was the loss of control over drinking activity, and the only possible treatment was total abstinence. His belief in this philosophy was so strong that he was spearheading a U.S. public education initiative to reduce public drunkenness The 1800s gave rise to the United States temperance movement. Alcohol was viewed as evil, the root cause of problems in America. Accepting the concept of alcoholism as a disease, people believed that liquor could enslave a person against his or her will. Proponents of temperance propagated the idea that drinking was so dangerous that people should not even try liquor, or that they would inevitably start on the road to alcoholism.

This philosophy maintained that alcohol is inherently dangerous for everyone and is inexorably addictive. We know today that there are strong genetic factors but not everyone is addicted to alcohol.

In the late 1800s, the temperance movement picked up steam and developed into a movement that promoted nationwide alcohol prohibition. According to advocates, the ban on alcohol will protect the family and eradicate sloth and spiritual degradation in the USA. Legislation was passed, supported by strong political powers, and prohibition went into effect in 1920.

Paradoxically, the prohibition era also marked the death of Victorian norms. Moving on from A. Sinclair in his book, Prohibition: The Age of Excess, a culture of liberated personal behavior developed and with it the notion that a full life should be followed by drinking. Drunkenness was personal liberty. Prohibition was abolished in 1933 due to public uproar.

<u>**The disease model of alcoholism**</u>

Alcoholics Anonymous (AA) was born shortly after prohibition ended. Formed in 1935 by stockbroker Bill Wilson and physicist Robert Smith, AA endorsed the idea that an alcoholic is unable to regulate his or her drinking, and that rehabilitation is only possible through total abstinence and peer support.

The key breakthrough in the theory of AA was that a biological explanation for alcoholism was suggested. A special group of alcoholics who are unable to regulate their drinking from birth was created. Initially, AA described this as "an addiction to alcohol." While AA was influential in re-emphasizing the "disease definition" of alcoholism, the defining work was done by the Yale Center of Alcohol Studies 'Elvin Jellinek, M.D. Jellinek described alcoholics as individuals with addiction, withdrawal symptoms and either "loss of control" or "incapacity to abstain" from alcohol in his book, The Disease Theory of Alcoholism, published 1960. He believed some individuals were unable to drink in moderation, and the disease became progressive and life-threatening with continued drinking.

Jellinek also recognized that cultural factors had influenced other aspects of the disease (e.g., failure to abstain and loss of control).

Numerous studies by behavioral and social scientists have backed Jellinek's argument about alcoholism as a disorder over the last 35 years. In 1957, the American Medical Association approved of the definition. Alcoholism is also listed as a disorder by the American Psychiatric Association, the American Medical Association, the American Public Health Association, the National Social Workers Association, the World Health Organization and the American College of Physicians.

However, the researchers ' results in the late 1970s led to clear requirements for an "alcohol dependence condition" now described in the Diagnostic and Statistical Manual of the[American Psychiatric Association] and the International Classification of Diseases of the World Health Organization.

The Joint Committee of the National Council on Alcoholism and Drug Dependence and the American Society of Addiction Medicine presented this concept for alcoholism in the 1992 Journal of the American Medical Association:

"Alcoholism is a primary chronic disease with genetic, psychosocial, and environmental factors affecting its nature and manifestations.

Often the disease is progressive, and terminal. It is characterized by impaired control over drinking, obsession with substance dependence, alcohol use despite adverse effects, and perception inconsistencies, often denials. Each of these signs can be chronic or intermittent.

3.2. Many Physicians still regard alcoholism as merely a bad behavior

Despite numerous studies validating the alcoholism model for the condition, there is still controversy. Social psychologist Stanton Peele, Ph.D., claims in his 1989 book, Diseasing of America, that AA and for-profit alcohol treatment facilities perpetuate the "myth" of alcoholism as a lifelong condition. He suggests that the idea of the disorder "excuses alcoholics for their past, present and future irresponsibility" and points out that most people are able to overcome addiction themselves.

He argues that the only effective response to alcoholism and other addictions is to "recreate living societies that cultivate the human capacity to lead productive lives." Ironically, Dr. Peele's belief that alcoholism is a question of personal conduct rather than a disorder tends to be more common among medical practitioners than among the general public.

A new Gallop poll found nearly 90% of Americans believe alcoholism is a disease. In comparison, the opinions of physicians on alcoholism were analyzed at an International Physicians of Alcoholics Anonymous (IDAA) conference held in August 1997. A scientific study published at that conference showed that 80 percent of responding doctors viewed alcoholism as pure bad behavior.

In in Lancet's November 1995 issue, Dr Raoul Walsh supports the claim that physicians have negative views regarding alcoholics. He cites empirical data showing that doctors appear to have negative views toward alcoholics, and that non-psychiatrists tend to view alcohol issues as predominantly psychiatrist concerns. He also claims that many doctors have negative attitudes towards patients with alcohol problems, since the majority of their clinical experience is dependent on late-stage alcohol.

Based on my experience in the field of addiction over the past 10 years, I conclude that many, if not most, health professionals still see alcohol addiction as a question of determination or behavior, and are resistant to seeing it as a disorder. Part of the problem is that medical schools provide little time to study alcoholism or addiction, and postgraduate training typically only deals with the end result of addiction or diseases related to alcohol / drugs.

Several studies conducted in the late 1980s provide evidence of insufficient knowledge of alcohol and alcohol issues among medical students and practitioners. Recent studies published in the Journal of Findings on Alcoholism also show that doctors do poorly in alcohol abuse diagnosis, prevention, and care.

Education is the single most important step to overcoming these obstacles.

Training must start at the undergraduate level, and continue throughout most, if not all, specialties ' preparation. This is particularly true for those in primary care where the most alcoholism problems are first seen. Promoting alcohol education programs in medical schools and at the postgraduate level has been improving in recent years.

For example, in Pennsylvania, most medical schools now offer at least one section of the curriculum on substance abuse. Medical specialty groups like the American Society of Addiction Medicine focus on increasing resident addiction training programs, practicing physicists and students.

As well as being available for in-house appointments, an increasing number of hospitals have an addiction medicine specialist on staff who is available for student and resident teaching.

The American Medical Association estimates that 25–40 per cent of patients in general hospital beds are there to treat alcohol-related ailments. The economic costs of alcohol abuse in the United States reach $115 billion per annum. Physicians in general practice, hospitals, and specialty medicine have tremendous potential to reduce the large burden of alcohol-related illness. For example, multiple randomized, controlled trials performed over the last few years show that brief physician interventions can significantly reduce the proportion of patients drinking at unsafe rates. But first, we do need to change our behaviors as physicians.

<u>Bio-psychosocial Disease</u>

Alcoholism should not be viewed as a willpower issue, abuse, or any other unscientific diagnosis. For what it is, the question must be accepted — a bio-psychosocial disorder with strong genetic effect, clear signs and symptoms, natural progression, and a fatal outcome unless treated. After 1988, the recognition of smoking as an addictive condition by the medical profession and the public has contributed to a decline in the use of nicotine in the United States. I feel that alcohol abuse will make similar strides.

As with smoking, we must begin by educating our own colleagues and reminding them that alcoholism is a disease. We must also emphasize that, through patient education, doctors have played a significant role in reducing mortality and morbidity from nicotine use. I think that we can achieve similar outcomes with alcohol abuse by effective physician involvement.

3.3. Addiction is a disease

The debate continues about whether alcohol or drug abuse is a disorder or not. Questions concerning the individual's responsibility for the disease and perception of brain pathophysiology are at the real core of this discussion.

Dorland's Medical Dictionary defines disease as "a definite morbid process with a typical train of symptoms; it can affect the entire body or any of its parts, and its etiology, anatomy, and prognosis may be known or unknown." The Jellinek curve graphically portrays the inexorable progression of debilitating symptoms from surreptitious use to compulsive use, to use amid adverse effects and subsequent alienation and loss of family, health, career and eventual incarceration or death.

The American Medical Association (AMA) declared in 1956 its view agreeing that alcoholism is a disease. And the AMA listed opioid addiction as a disease in 1987. In its International Classification of Diseases, Volume Ten (ICD-X), the World Health Organization lists the chemical dependency among other disorders. In the Diagnostic and Statistical Manual, Volume Four (DSM-IV), most medical professional organizations consider addiction a disease, including the American Psychiatric Association which lists drug dependency criteria along with other mental disorders.

So, where is the argument, if all these official bodies have accepted that addiction is a disease? This arrives, oddly enough, from the general public, media commentators and law enforcement agencies.

Many people have a mistaken view of the disease as something that invades or threatens your good health; an innocent victim targeted by a "perpetrator" who has no power over him or her. The disease theory isn't right with addiction. And it is here that the dispute starts. In addition, the individual is involved in or induces many of their own behavioral problems.

Most illnesses are potentially, at least in part, self-imposed by behavior. If someone smokes cigarettes and consumes fatty foods, and has coronary artery disease, they have developed their own problem to a large extent.

Similarly, someone with a diabetes family history who eats enough to get overweight and then develops diabetes has defied fate and caused much of their own problem. We are a victim of their own inappropriate behavior. It's not that they preferred to have heart disease or diabetes, but rather they unintentionally chose habits that have undesirable consequences in pursuit of their chosen lifestyle. Likewise, when someone drinks it's never their intention to become addicted; however, their action has created their own problem, in part, and largely in ignorance.

The fact that addiction is a disorder should not eliminate the burden of responsibility for cause (at least in part) or care in any way. Addiction is like many other illnesses, in this sense.

There's no clear precise pathophysiology of addiction. Possible causal explanations include irregular or specific neurotransmitter receptors such as dopamine or serotonin, various neuroanatomic interactions or different chemical responses to addictive drugs. If the exact deficiency were identified it would be much easier to accept the addiction as a disease. Of example, if addiction was induced by a mutated dopamine gene structure called the A1 allele, then we could call addiction the "dopamine A1 allele disorder." It is difficult to understand and diagnose because we don't know the pathophysiology with certainty.

Numerous conceptual models for understanding addiction have been identified by Hester and Miller. We also list moral, temperance, ethical, educational, financial, biological, genetic, sociocultural, general structures, and public health models, including the dispositional disease model. All of these models have validity and draw attention to different facets of the dynamic addiction problem.

Again addiction is like other diseases in this way. Different models exist for understanding coronary artery disease, for example. Much has been said about personality type A and B with coronary disease as leading or preventive to the disease. There are also social educational factors associated with heart disease. Heredity and diet are important factors as are lifestyle problems, fitness issues and self-care issues. There is a genetic viewpoint, and also a biological one.

There is even a moral model of heart disease as the primary cause of the problem, focusing on gluttony and/or "bad habits." It is also not clear the exact cause of coronary disease.

3.4. Addicts do bad things

Unlike most other disorders, addiction is one way.   The abusers do bad things in the wake of their disease. They lie, they steal, they cheat and they are unreliable.
Ultimately the temptation to use overcomes moral constraints. The temptation to use is in excess of principles. The desire to use is so powerful that it goes beyond most other drives. Addicts are doing bad things and they should be accountable and expect consequences. This does not mean however that addiction is not a disorder.

The fact that AIDS patients are willing to steal drugs to buy doesn't mean that AIDS isn't a disease. The fact that promiscuity contributes to diseases that are sexually transmitted does not mean syphilis is not a problem.

Addiction is something of a disorder. Comprehension of this reality supports patients and families. Such awareness helps the patient get less shame and guilt and start a process of acceptance of support. In diminishing their anger and frustration, the family benefits and they begin to support safe recovery programs and care for the patient and themselves.

Chapter 4: Alcoholism Has Genetic Basis

It seems clear that, once drug use has started, not everyone brings the same degree of risk to experience serious, persistent issues. That argument is really no different from what one would expect for most medical disorders, since different individuals tend to be carrying higher or lower rates of susceptibility to heart attacks, cancer, obesity, etc. Many people believe that different levels of susceptibility to developing alcohol or drug dependency are due to biological differences that exist between individuals, at least in part.

4.1. The important genetic factors

Over the past twenty years, most of my work has centered on one significant form of biological factor that could lead to different levels of susceptibility to serious substance-related problems. That is the potential role genetics may play in developing alcohol dependence or alcoholism. By this I mean the way in which the biological material or genes transmitted from parents to children can predispose someone to a higher or lower vulnerability to serious and repeated problems related to alcohol.

Sadly, genetic influences linked to dependency on other substances such as stimulants, marijuana-type narcotics, or opiates are less understood but new and interesting data are now being developed even here. Though, since I want to keep my main focus on what's real (rather than what's expected to be), I have to restrict the remarks that are mostly given here to alcohol.

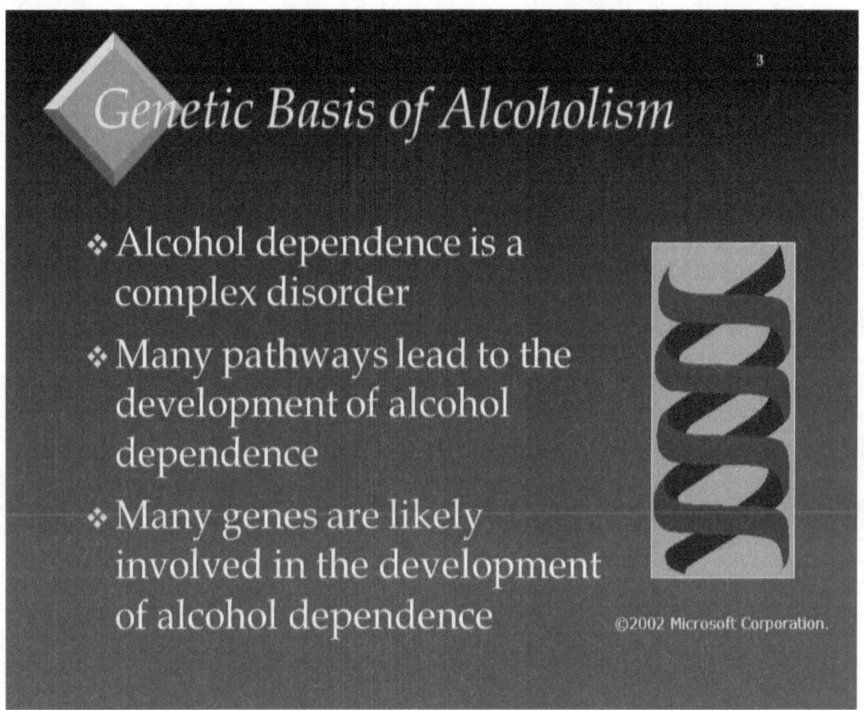

It has been acknowledged for hundreds of years that alcoholism runs deeply within families. Nevertheless, until relatively recently, most believed that the double to fourfold increased risk of severe alcohol problems among close alcoholic relatives was a consequence of the family environment in which people were brought up. For example, a child raised in a home where heavy drinking was the norm might be expected to believe that alcohol is a way to deal with problems.

According to this hypothesis, a person like that could be expected to develop more alcohol-related problems later in life than someone raised in a home where drunkenness was frowned on and alcohol was consumed in only moderate amounts or not at all. Studies conducted in the 1960s, however, began to question this presumption regarding the all-important role of environmental factors in alcohol production.

4.2. Research studies of twins and adopted children of alcoholics

The first form of study to start testing the relative importance of the twin-focused genetics versus childhood. Here, researchers benefitted from the fact that nature produces two forms of twins.At the same time, fraternal twins are born but share just 50 percent of their chromosomes, just like any other brothers and sisters. We come from different eggs and sperm whilst at the same time implanting two separate fertilized eggs in the womb. On the other hand, identical twins are also born together, but they actually share 100 per cent of their chromosomes. They come from the same fertilized egg, which after multiple divisions splits up into two separate individuals.

All forms of twin sets are born in the same setting and undergo significant childhood experiences at the same age and under the same general conditions of life. Therefore, if severe alcohol-related life issues were the result of major events occurring in childhood (i.e. environmental influences), then an alcoholic's twin should be at a very high risk for the disorder himself or herself, regardless of whether it involves fraternal or identical twinning.

On the other hand, if genetic factors are significant, an alcoholic's identical twin, sharing 100 percent of the genes, should be at a much higher risk than a fraternal twin for developing this problem. Almost all of the research carried out in this field over the last twenty years show that the risk of alcoholism is much higher in an alcoholic's identical twin (maybe as high as 60 percent) than in the fraternal twins (estimated at 30%). Such results support the belief that genetic factors play a significant role in assessing the alcohol risk.

Nevertheless, to me the most convincing evidence about the role of genetic factors in alcoholism comes from research of children of alcoholics who have been adopted away from birth. Here one may assess the risk of alcoholism among alcoholic biological children raised by non-alcoholics. It is amazing because even though they had no idea that their biological parent had alcoholism, these sons and daughters nevertheless show their fourfold increased risk for severe alcohol issues. Nevertheless, even if one of the adoptive parents of the children develops alcoholism, this does not raise the risk of alcoholism for the adopted child any more than is expected by the question of the biological parent.

In other words, the condition in the biological parent indicates a high risk for severe alcohol issues, not problems in the setting in which the child is born. The discovery that genetic factors influence alcoholism doesn't mean that genes alone cause severe alcohol problems. Many environmental factors must also play a role because even an alcoholic's identical twin is never as high as 100 percent at risk of the condition. In other words, no one is predestined to become an alcoholic, and no one has a 100% chance for cancer or heart disease to grow.

And even though we have a higher risk of developing serious and chronic alcohol-related problems, we still have options as to what we are doing about it.

We are the ones who decide whether we're going to drink at all, and we each assess the steps we take to avoid drunkenness, the way we restrict drinking in times of stress, and whether the creation of more minor problems can cause us to continue using alcohol and stop putting ourselves in risk.

4.3. Alcoholics must not be blamed for their disease

How would you react if a loved one were diagnosed with cancer, or diabetes, or mental illness such as schizophrenia or manic-depression?

Alcoholism is a disease which is no different from cancer, or diabetes, or mental disorders with various forms of treatment available and different levels of success with successful treatment. Alcoholism is a disease of the biological brains. If alcohol or other addictive drugs are injected into a body predisposed to addiction through inherited biology, there are irreversible biological changes in the brain. Without the genetic predisposition to addiction such modifications do not occur in anyone.

We are all born with "predispositions" that are hereditary with an increased chance, based on our ancestry, of having such physical or mental disorders during our lifetime. If the family side of the mother has members who have been diagnosed with cancer, or the family side of the father has members who have been diagnosed with heart disease or diabetes, there is an increased risk for the child at some point in life to manifest one of those diseases.

Genetics have a part to play in disease development. Emotional and environmental factors all need to work together to establish illness. Possession of a portion of the sum doesn't make a whole. Knowledge of the predisposing factors is only markers, not an inevitable fate.

When all the parts come together to manifest the whole and the disorder, there is a particular fate for people suffering from alcohol disease that usually does not occur when there is any other disease. It is to be blamed for their illness as if the illness is a sign of weakness, moral failure or lack of sufficient willpower and internal control to handle addiction.

Cruelty vs. compassion

Blaming someone for their addiction is unimaginably cruel and yet alcoholics are blamed for causing their disease because alcoholism is considered a lifestyle choice.

When diagnosing almost any other illness, effective types of treatment options are explored. Odds are issued on remission. One out of 10. Five out of 10. The emphasis is on' one out of ten' or' one out of five.' It doesn't matter how long it takes for the medical treatments or how long and windy the road to recovery is. Setbacks are seen as a challenge for more commitment to recovery. Loved ones never let go, friends with constructive reinforcement rally around and some employers will change work schedules to protect your place with the organization.

When the condition is intoxication it should not be otherwise.

Initial treatment for alcoholism and drug addictions usually involves admission to an alcoholism and drug addiction-specific inpatient / outpatient treatment facility. There is a phase of detoxification, accompanied by therapy, schooling, support groups and meetings in 12 steps. Most treatment centers have a family plan in which the family members are interested in rehabilitation.

The treatment center is a starting point of recuperation life.

Continued abstinence from alcohol approaches the physical; support group therapy and engagement discusses the social, mental, and spiritual.

Recovery, as with any disease, is not always a straight road to success.

Remission times and potential relapse may occur. If a relapse occurs, measured as a temporary setback rather than a failure, with the challenge of modifying or enhancing the treatment course in an effort to find a workable mix, then recovery is likely to continue. This would be the possibility if the treatment for cancer, diabetes or a mental disorder did not bring results hoped for.

When the condition is intoxication it should not be otherwise.

Chapter 5: The Genesis Of Cure For Alcoholism

I Will QUIT when I want. I am not addicted; I just enjoy drinking. How often did you say those words to yourself or to those around you? Okay, maybe you're not addicted but you can't even stop. You're in the middle somewhere. You know that drinking too much alcohol is dangerous to your health, you know you're drinking too much at times and doing things you wish you didn't have, and you know that the hangovers are getting worse.

But you also know it would be too hard for you to leave the "cold turkey" and never drink again; you think it would be a nightmare. You don't think it is any other way.

5.1. Sinclair discovers what drives alcoholism

Who would have thought that a little boy taunted on a school bus in West Virginia for having a speech impediment would one day crack the code behind a bewildering epidemic that kills 1.8 million people every year, according to the World Health Organization?

Sinclair's "right brain" behaviors were promoted at the same time when most people could not grasp what he said. His sketches were comparable to those twice his age made by the students.

He was admitted into art classes in the local college at the age of eleven. He was appointed the "Official Artist of the School" by his grade school teacher, mostly to inspire him to hang around and at least learn how to read and write. He began to catch up academically with his peculiar aptitude for visual and spatial concepts, and eventually graduated at the top of his class. He also resolved his struggle with expression and is remembered today for his ability to speak eloquently about abstract ideas.

Sinclair subsequently received scholarships at the Carnegie Institute of Technology in Pennsylvania in 1961 to study physics. Carnegie at that time had one of the first computers, the BendixG-20, fitted with 32,000 vacuum tubes. That is about half of my cell phone's power, but it was a wonder for its day; Sinclair's experience with it had a profound influence on his later neuroscience research. You can't just draw in a black box marked with reward or punishment while programming a computer; you have to describe exactly how this process works.

On the other hand, the discovery of the complex "behavior" that the G-20 might produce with pure wires and vacuum tubes led Sinclair to believe that the physical foundation for our own human behavior might be understandable.

Sinclair's curiosity in behavior has led him to study into alcohol, first at Cincinnati University and then at Oregon University.

His discovery of the Alcohol Deprivation Effect (ADE) was a significant, but largely accidental, factor.7 The ADE proved to be the first step in breaking the alcohol addiction code.

Dr. R. J. Senter had an alcohol research grant at the University of Cincinnati, and in 1964 he recruited Sinclair as an enthusiastic undergraduate student to help care for laboratory rat. At the time, the common assumption was that rats and other animals did not like alcohol, and thus were not relevant to human alcoholism research. And that was basically what they discovered at Cincinnati. The rats had a choice of two bottles they could drink from, one filled with water and the other filled with an alcohol solution. The rats took about 70 percent of their water bottle volume, and only about 30 percent from the bottle of alcohol.

Rat had seemed to prefer alcohol to water.

Sinclair had an idea for his own experiment, and asked Senter if he might have rats. Senter agreed but said that he would have to use animals that were used as controls in an earlier study because there was no additional animal funding. The rats had been given a choice between water and alcohol over several weeks in the previous experiment. Those rats were left in their cages for a few weeks at the end of that experiment with free access to food and water but no alcohol.

It was then that Sinclair first made a potential discovery that would have major ramifications for studies into the causes of alcoholism in humans and ultimate cure. It must have come as bold a discovery as Isaac Newton's when he observed an apple falling from a tree — an observation that is said to have caused the development of the principle of universal gravitation in Newtonian physics — in evoking an entirely new way of understanding the mechanisms driving addiction.

Sinclair recounts what happened: So, as rats usually sleep in the middle of the afternoon, I went down to the rat room and started placing alcohol bottles back on the cages. To my surprise, the rats suddenly woke up, came to the front of the cage and started drinking vigorously with the alcohol solution.

They paid no attention to the bottle of water beside it. Their appetite for alcohol slowly returned to normal levels over the next week, but I could have no doubt that these rats had shown a high desire for alcohol, having seen that high level of consumption when the alcohol first returned. (Sinclair, 1997) The Alcohol Deprivation Effect (ADE) has proved to be one of the most strong and efficient factors regulating alcohol consumption.

It is still one of the most researched effects of drug research today, fourty years later. The findings from these studies have shown conclusively that abstinence from alcohol in rats used to drink also increases their appetite for alcohol. This is not only occurring in rats and other animals but also in humans. The idea was that the more deprived an alcoholic is of alcohol, the more likely he is to desire it.

Since the 1968 publication of the paper describing the impact of alcohol deprivation, recognizing why alcoholism and many other addictions are becoming living conditions has become recognized as important. First of all, it's important to drink alcohol regularly for a long time— in rats for several weeks — to develop an alcohol addiction.

After that, as T-k Li, the National Institute on Alcohol Abuse and Alcoholism (NIAAA) CEO, has said, alcohol motivation is purely a matter of scheduling. It's similar to the food and water inspiration. If you want to research hunger after the Thanksgiving meal, you are not looking for it immediately. You look at those people who have gone without feeding for many hours or days. Likewise, if you want to see high alcohol motivation, you're researching rats or people who have been deprived of it for weeks.

When the alcohol is first retrieved the desire for alcohol is most clearly seen. The rats are unable to tell you they are starving for a beer, but as soon as you reopen the bar by putting their alcohol bottles back on their cages, they immediately start drinking enthusiastically again. During the first few minutes after the conclusion of the deprivation, the rate of alcohol consumption is more than fifteen times the amount seen daily without deprivation. Once the initial binge drinking in deprived alcoholic rats has run its course, they return to their previous levels. The effect of alcohol-deprivation is not only seen in animals but also in human alcoholics.

The curves show how addiction increases over time when alcoholics— rats or humans — are deprived of alcohol, and how they binge when they gain access. The ADE has significant medical effects. Typical drug treatment has been detoxification followed by weeks of forced abstinence. The ADE suggests that forced abstinence is not a treatment which is successful. It does not cure alcoholism but, in addition, causes an increase in cravings which helps to produce relapses. Recently, the National Institute on Drug Abuse (NIDA) found an association with cocaine that is close to the ADE; the director, Nora D. Volkow, pointed out that it shows that incarceration alone is not an appropriate treatment for cocaine abuse, either.

The ADE describes how alcoholics who are already addicted are continually seeking alcohol when they abstain from alcohol for a period of time.

The deprivation or abstinence can result from incarceration or hospitalization. The isolation is often self-imposed through abstinence-based or faith-based approaches such as Alcoholics Anonymous, which enable members to hire a Higher Power to help them stay dry "one day at a time." Many treatments often rely on abstinence and the use of willpower to go cold Turkish.

Sinclair's findings and all the ADE studies that accompanied it prove that abstinence does not eradicate alcohol cravings, and therefore why abstinence is not a successful treatment for the vast majority of people.

The ADE also has important theoretical consequences for the causes of dependency. The prevalent view at the time of discovery of the ADE was that alcoholism was caused by physiological alcohol dependence. It was already evident to the experts of the day that the enjoyment created by alcohol could not justify the alcohol abuse. Many alcoholics report having very little if any satisfaction at all. Perhaps drinking alcohol was fun at one time, but not when it reached the stage of alcoholism— clearly, whatever leftovers of enjoyment remained was inadequate to offset all the pain and suffering they knew their drinking alcohol caused. But they continued drinking once they were hooked.

The theory arose to clarify this disparity that the reason alcoholics drank was to avoid, or stop, the very negative effects of alcohol withdrawal. This theory created the theoretical ambiguity that we still have today: alcoholism is considered "alcohol dependency," but that doesn't mean alcoholism is a pure physiological dependence that the body produces when it adapts to the sustained presence of alcohol.

This theory has also been one of the reasons for the usual treatment. It was hoped that the primary reason for drinking would be eliminated once the alcoholics had been taken through the painful process of withdrawal — had been subjected to detoxification. Nonetheless, if alcohol dependency (meaning alcoholism) were induced by alcohol dependence (meaning physiological dependence created by adaptation), the solution would have been detoxification.

The ADE has shown that physiological dependency isn't necessary for drinking motivation. Only a few days of abstinence reverses a basic physiological dependency. However, when the dependency is removed the desire for alcohol in animals that have learned to drink does not go away, but instead increases.

In fact, the timeframe for it to rise varies from the withdrawal time frame.

5.2. Learning and reinforcement

Sinclair built on the early experiments of Ivan Pavlov, the Russian physiologist who was awarded the 1904 Nobel Prize for his work on the understanding and extinguishing of behaviors.

Pavlov's famous experiments showed how dogs learned to salivate when a bell rung, because before the dogs were given food (reinforcement) the bell had been rung. Training depends on the dog being rewarded with food whenever it sounds like a bell. Once the behavior was conditioned, and the dog was salivating at the bell's sound, Pavlov rang the bell, but gave no food. Eventually, each time the bell was heard, the dog was slowly salivating less. Pavlov stopped his brain from receiving positive reinforcement by not feeding the dog food when the bell was being rang.

Every time this happened, the dog's nervous system responded by undermining the action it had previously learned. Less and less saliva was developed and finally none at the sound of the bell was released. This mechanism has been named extinction — a deceptively simple and especially powerful biological mechanism to reverse learned behavior.

Extinction doesn't just know the bell doesn't mean food any more. Extinction is a separate learning process which obeys different rules.13 For example, learning works best when there's plenty of time between each trial, but extinction involves "massed trials." If Pavlov had only rung the bell once a week without giving food, there would have been little or no reduction in salivation rates. Then, in a short time, he had to ring it over and over again.

Experiments with genetically predisposed AA rats to become addicted led Sinclair to the belief that the drug problem was acquired and can be eliminated through extinction. He knew extinction happens when a response is given but the required strengthening is blocked. So the problem is, how can the reinforcement be blocked? How can you drink alcohol with a rat or human, taste it, feel the intoxication but still not get the reinforcement? Unless Sinclair could figure out a way to do this, the excessive drinking could be extinguished and the epidemic fixed.

Nevertheless, in order to answer this question it was necessary to know how alcohol gives rise to strengthening. The response was indicated by the work Sinclair had already started back in Oregon on the influence of morphine on alcohol drinking. If morphine meets the need for alcohol (and alcohol satisfies the need for opiates), then both medications are likely to produce reinforcement in the same manner. Scientific evidence has shown that morphine and other opiate drugs (such as heroin) have created their addictive or reinforcing effects by binding to specific receptors in the brain, called opioid receptors.

Obviously the brain did not develop opioid receptors for binding opium poppy extracts. As soon as it was discovered, the body has its endogenous opioids, called endorphins, which are the natural substance that binds to opioid receptors. * The reason why cocaine, heroin, morphine, and other opioids will affect the brain is that these drugs all have endorphin-like molecular shapes and thus, like endorphins, may attach and trigger the opioid receptors. Sinclair found that preventing the opioid receptors in the brain from connecting with the endorphins produced each time alcohol is consumed would be the way to do this.

The next step was to find a way to do that.

Fortunately for Sinclair, the methods already existed for getting inside the brain to suppress the endorphins, in the form of compounds called opioid antagonists. These are medications that actually block opiates, such as morphine or methamphetamine, and cannabinoids, such as endorphins, from connecting the brain to the opioid receptors.

 Such medications had been around since the early 1960s. * * ** In taking advantage of these drugs ' ability to block the effects of endorphins, Sinclair was to launch the most effective substance re-search effort— the elimination of alcohol addictions.

Sinclair's opioid-blocking or antagonistic drugs used to facilitate the de-addiction process were short-acting naloxone and its longer-acting equivalents, naltrexone and nalmefene.

Opioid antagonists have long been used to reverse the effects of opiates such as morphine in routine anesthesia. Opioid antagonists have the ability to block opioid receptors from recognizing opioids within the brain. Sinclair uses the analogy to put the wrong key inside a lock. As long as naltrexone is in the endorphin-designed lock, endorphin itself and other opiates bounce off and have no effect; at the same time, naltrexone itself is the wrong key, and cannot unlock the lock.

In other words, once the body has consumed opioid antagonistic drugs such as naltrexone, the opioid pathway in the brain is locked down. The endorphins therefore cannot activate or inhibit opioid receptors in the brain.

Opioid antagonists have no other effects, and do not make you feel high or low. Yet they're so strong they can reverse the effects of opiates in the brain even if you've already had an overdose of opiates. The short-acting opioid antagonist naloxone is currently used as a life-saving treatment in hospitals around the world to reverse the effects of narcotic addiction from heroin overdoses.

5.3. De-addiction and cure

Sinclair performed dozens of studies on naltrexone, nalmefene, and naloxone on the high-drinking line of AA rats and other animals already addicted to alcohol before carrying out the clinical trials on humans. Sinclair's experiments showed that the animals decreased their consumption of the alcohol solution when addicted rats were given the antagonist to block the opioid (endorphin) receptors within their brains. That was an important finding as it meant the drugs would benefit alcoholics too.

However, just as significant was the trend of how drinking decreased because that demonstrated the process by which the antagonists function, and therefore the manner in which the drugs should be used by humans.

Typical experiment findings are shown in Figure 2. The rats had been drinking alcohol solution for many weeks and now only got it one hour a day — a kind of "happy hour." They had water and food available all the time, but every day the rats would hurry up and start drinking intensely, due to the Alcohol Deprivation Effect, when the alcohol bottles were put on the cages. The first bar shows the average amount of alcohol they have drank during the week before treatment in every happy hour.

The rats then had administered an antagonist drug (in this case nalmefene) shortly before each of the next five daily sessions. Remember that alcohol consumption during the first session was not reduced; rather, the drinking on the first day of therapy was slightly higher in this experiment.

That is very significant. The drug itself did not relieve the cravings of rats. When the bottles of alcohol were put on the cages, the rats all came running up to the front of the cage and started drinking quickly.

The drug had no effect until after the rats consumed the alcohol, the alcohol was ingested and gone into the brain, and endorphins released. The medication blocked the endorphin effect at that point— it blocked the anticipated positive reinforcement usually provided by the endorphins.

As a result of this effect, the alcohol drinking activity and the appetite for it were somewhat diminished by the extinction mechanism. That only comes up on the second day of treatment for the first time. This time the rats were slower in coming to the bottles when alcohol was offered, and they drank substantially less of it. However, after that alcohol was consumed and endorphins were released, the reinforcement was blocked by the medication once more. Consequently the conduct was further impaired so the rats showed even less interest in alcohol on the third day. Every day that alcohol was consumed and encouragement was not sought was yet another extinction experiment that further undermined drinking and cravings. By the fifth day, during the not - so-happy hour, just one of the rats bothered to come up to the alcohol jar.

The next day in the chart, called "Post 1," the rats were given no antagonisms before they had access to alcohol. Almost all of the previous day's drugs should have been removed but very little alcohol was still consumed by the rats. The next court, "Post 2," was one week later, when the adversary would certainly have gone away from their systems, but the drinking was still significantly reduced. That is important too. Once again, it indicates that it was not the drug itself that decreased alcohol consumption; the medication was gone, but the drinking was still diminished. Then, the combination of drinking while on the drug— Naltrexone + Drinking — had disrupted the cabling in the brains of rats that induces drinking and cravings.

Note, however, that the post-day drinking is back up. On these days when no adversary was given and alcohol was consumed it again provided reinforcement and relearned the drinking activity. It came as no surprise because extinct habits are considered to be easily re-learnable.

The addicted animals stopped drinking, because after drinking the antagonist blocked endorphin reinforcement.

Sinclair named this pharmacological extinction de-addiction technique, which has now become known as the Sinclair method.* Sinclair clearly showed that extinction was responsible for the reduction of excessive drinking. He went on to replicate these experiments in every way he could imagine. The same trend of reduced consumption for alcohol and saccharin was always found, both of which produce endorphins in the brain. However, when used properly, opioid antagonist drugs reduce the intake of other substances, such as opioid methadone, which is close to morphine. ** Learning and extinction curves are equivalent in rats and humans, except that extinction occurs faster in rats who have learned to drink in just one laboratory setting than in humans who have learned to drink for a year.

5.4. Reduction in craving with Real Patients

External triggers (such as seeing a bottle of wine or passing a bar) and internal triggers (such as self-drinking thoughts and photos, or certain mood conditions, such as feeling in party mood or feeling depressed) that cause the urge to drink.

Physiologically speaking, they trigger certain neuronal pathways to fire, and when these neurons fire, the person experiences an alcohol craving. If these neurons fire enough, then the person begins to drink.

Once alcohol is absorbed into the bloodstream and then transferred to the nervous system, it causes the release of endorphins.

The endorphin molecules, like a local hormone, circulate around the brain and bind to the opioid receptors. It stimulates the receptors, allowing them to reinforce neuronal pathways that had just been used. The route that had just been used in this case is the one that triggers intoxication, and the symptoms of alcohol addiction. The more this happens, the clearer it becomes the receptors that trigger drinking and craving.

Getting reinforced makes it easier for those neurons to fire in the future. Firstly, it is impossible that the sight of a wine bottle or the feeling of being in party mood can make people think of alcohol, and rarely make them drink. But, after many drinking sessions have reinforced the neuron route, when people are again in the same situation, they want to drink, and actually do so.

After many months and years of drinking and getting reinforced by endorphins, the receptors that generate all the alcohol-related habits are permanently hard-wired into the brain. After reaching this point, humans have little or no control over drinking; they have become addicted to alcohol.

Alcohol consumption leads to addiction even faster if there is a genetic predisposition to alcoholism. It is possible without the "right" genetic predisposition but doubtful somebody will ever develop a drinking problem. But people with the "right" hereditary alcohol makeup won't become addicted if they never drink in the first place.

The pathways in the brain that generate alcohol will eventually expand into "super-highways" in those who have developed the ability to become addicted and drink. When learned over years of drinking, these super-highways remain open to life, never inactive or disappearing. You are with someone forever, which is why abstinence is so difficult for alcoholics. Regardless of which secular or spiritual therapy they accept, most alcoholics will relapse within months of starting their treatment. Alcoholics Anonymous states: "Once an alcoholic, always an alcoholic." Alcoholism is a permanent condition— unless and until it can be separated from the addictive neural pathways that regulate it.

Fortunately, these toxic hard-wired nerve pathways can now be deleted throughout the brain. If these superhighways are phased out, the abuse is reversed. Sinclair has managed to show that this method of de-addiction can be accomplished through the pharmacological withdrawal cycle, which is made possible by the use of naltrexone to inhibit the stimulation of endorphins released into the brain each time someone drinks. Pharmacological treatment for elimination includes the combination of Naltrexone + drinking to reverse the over-reinforced alcohol-drinking mechanism and slowly return it to its earlier, pre-addicted state. The pharmacological withdrawal process happens slowly and incrementally each time alcohol is consumed when naltrexone in one's body inhibits endorphin activity on opioid receptors in the brain. The super-highways are cut back, and once again become one-lane country roads.

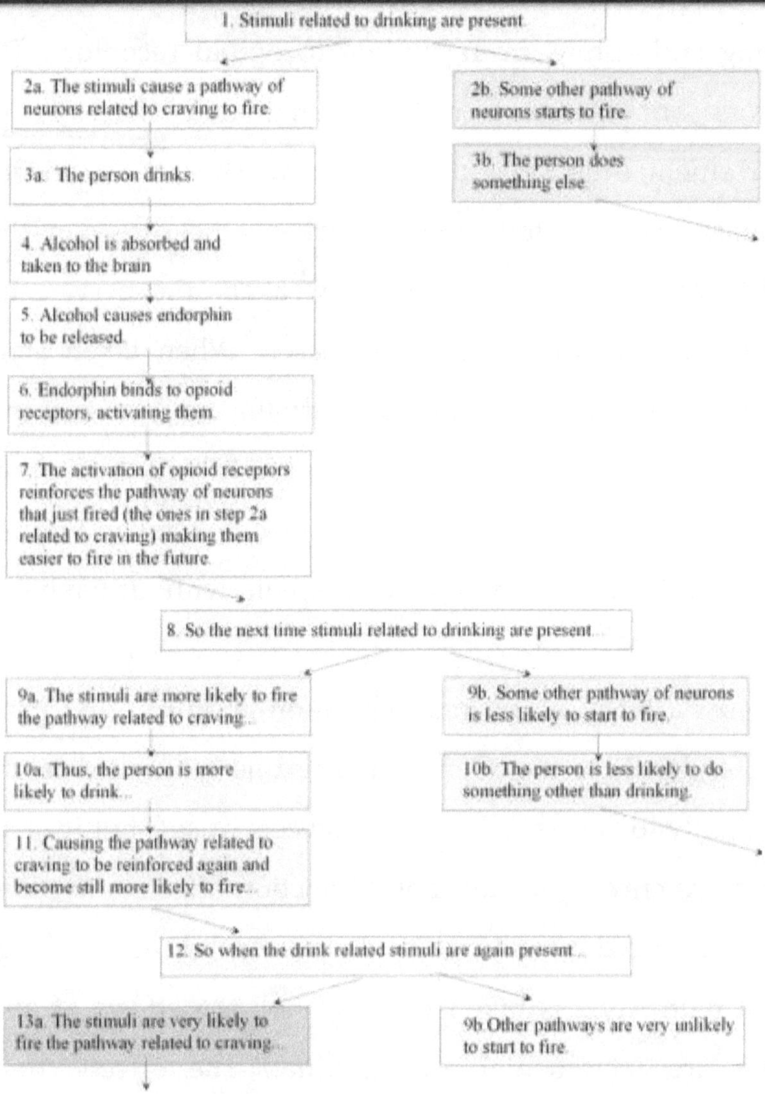

1. Stimuli related to drinking are present.

2a. The stimuli cause a pathway of neurons related to craving to fire.

2b. Some other pathway of neurons starts to fire.

3a. The person drinks.

3b. The person does something else.

4. Alcohol is absorbed and taken to the brain

5. Alcohol causes endorphin to be released.

6. Endorphin binds to opioid receptors, activating them.

7. The activation of opioid receptors reinforces the pathway of neurons that just fired (the ones in step 2a related to craving) making them easier to fire in the future.

8. So the next time stimuli related to drinking are present...

9a. The stimuli are more likely to fire the pathway related to craving...

9b. Some other pathway of neurons is less likely to start to fire.

10a. Thus, the person is more likely to drink...

10b. The person is less likely to do something other than drinking.

11. Causing the pathway related to craving to be reinforced again and become still more likely to fire...

12. So when the drink related stimuli are again present...

13a. The stimuli are very likely to fire the pathway related to craving...

9b Other pathways are very unlikely to start to fire.

Naltrexone works at Step 6 as illustrated in Figure above, stopping endorphins from binding to opioid receptors. The receptors are therefore not activated and there is no reinforcement; thus Step 7 does not occur. Then, the extinction mechanism is activated, which weakens the direction that failed to provide reinforcement. It weakens the nerves that cause desire and drinking in this case. When taken alone without smoking, naltrexone has virtually no "anti-craving" effects. If one does not drink alcohol it will not pump endorphins into the brain. When naltrexone is taken without eating, it just stays on the opioid receptors without having to block it.

That's just a bit of an oversimplification because other items trigger endorphins too. Getting naltrexone without drinking may slightly lower one's interest in sweets or sex, but it won't lower one's craving for alcohol. Extinction affects only those activities induced by endorphins that arise while on the drug. Even if naltrexone is taken with alcohol, the effects of anti-craving are incremental and gradual. The effects aren't necessarily seen in actual alcoholics.

Chapter 6: Treatment Of Alcoholism

The first step in rehabilitation is understanding that there is a question with drug dependency.

The next move is to reach out for support. This is available from a number of community networks and specialist resources.

6.1. Recovery methods

Recognized recovery methods for alcoholism are the following:

Do-it-yourself: Certain individuals with an alcohol addiction tend to minimize or abstain without obtaining medical assistance. Websites offer free information, and self-help books can be purchased online.

Counseling: A trained psychologist may help the client discuss his or her issues and then formulate a recovery strategy. Cognitive behavioral therapy (CBT) is commonly used for the treatment of drug dependency.

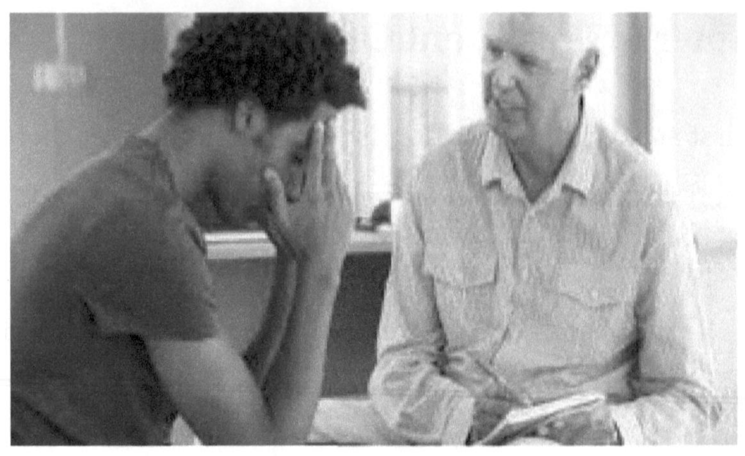

Treatment of underlying problems: self-esteem, stress, anxiety, depression or other mental health issues can occur. Because they will raise the risks posed by alcohol, it is necessary to address these issues too. Popular conditions linked to drinking, such as obesity, liver disease and likely heart disease, will also need to be treated.

Rehabilitation programs: they may include specialist medical help, individual or group counseling, support services, instruction, social engagement, intervention counseling and a variety of substance dependency recovery approaches. It is good for certain people to be physically free from the exposure to temptation.

A drug that triggers a serious alcohol reaction: Antabuse (disulfiram) induces an extreme reaction while someone is consuming alcohol, causing diarrhea, flushing, vomiting and headaches. It's a deterrent but in the long run it won't address the urge to drink or fix the problems

Craving drugs: Naltrexone (ReVia) can help to minimize the desire to have a drink. Acamprosate (Campral) can aid in cravings.

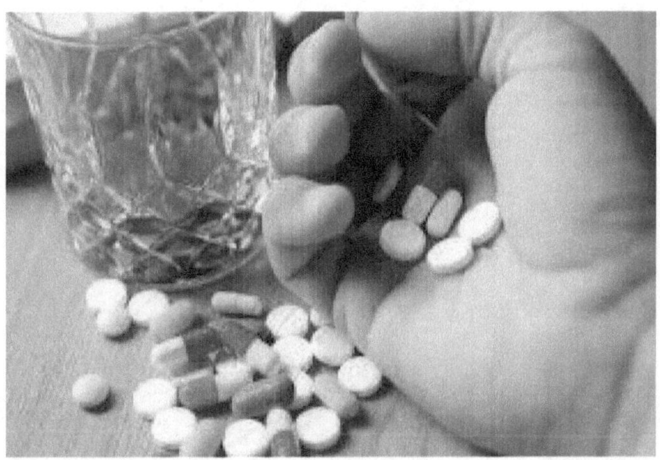

Detoxification: medications may help avoid signs of withdrawal (delirium tremors, or DTs) that could occur after leaving. Treatment normally lasts from 4 to 7 days. Chlordiazepoxide, a benzodiazepine drug, is also used for detoxification (detoxification).

Abstinence: Many people successfully achieve abstinence, but shortly after or many time after they start drinking again. Entry to therapy, medical care, support services and support for the family will all help the patient escape alcohol as time goes by.

Alcoholics Anonymous: Anonymous Alcoholics is a voluntary association of men and women facing alcohol issues. It is non-professional, self-supporting, multiracial, apolitical and virtually anywhere available. There are no requirements for age, or education. Membership is open to anybody who would like to stop drinking.

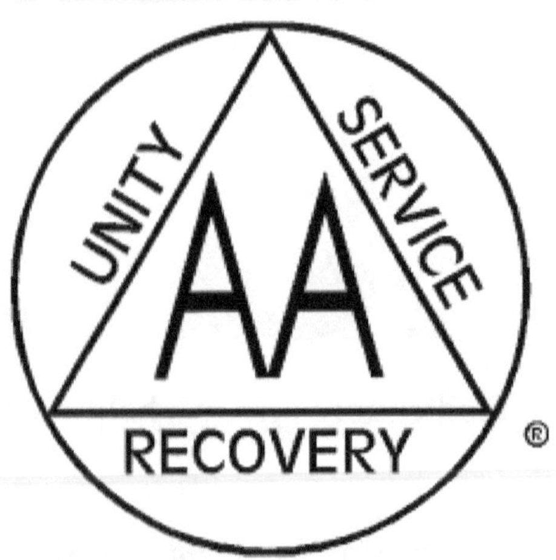

Therapeutic Therapies: Also known as drug therapy, therapeutic therapies include working with a health care provider to identify habits that contribute to heavy drinking to make them improve. Behavioral therapies have similar features, which may include:

- Developing the techniques required to discourage or decrease alcohol

- Helping to develop a healthy social support network

- Moving towards realistic targets

- Addressing or preventing causes that can induce relapse Examples of Behavioral Therapies

Cognitive–Behavioral Therapy that work one-on - one with a psychiatrist or in limited g. The aim of this type of treatment is to recognize the emotions and circumstances (called "cues") that contribute to excessive drinking and stress control that could contribute to relapse. The aim is to improve the patterns of thought that lead to binge drinking, and to build the skills required to deal with daily circumstances that that cause drinking issues.

Motivational Training Treatment takes place in a brief amount of time to develop and enhance encouragement for improving drinking behavior. The counseling focused on understanding the benefits and cons of seeking care, creating a strategy to improve one's alcohol, establishing faith, and learning the skills needed to contribute to the program.

In the recovery process, marriage and social counselling includes partners and other family members and may play a significant part in the reparation and strengthening of family ties. Studies suggest that good family involvement by family therapy improves abstinence (stop drinking) chances relative to adult counseling patients.

Specific treatments are brief, time-limited, one-on - one or small group therapy sessions. The psychologist offers details about the drinking habit and possible consequences for the patient. The psychologist will meet with the client after providing individual input to set expectations and offer suggestions for helping create a difference. Essentially, opting to seek help can be more relevant than the solution chosen, as long as the solution prevents harsh debate which provides empathy, motivational encouragement and an emphasis on improving drinking behavior.

6.2. When is the time of treatment?

Alcohol-related problems— which arise from drinking too much, too much, or too frequently — are among the most important public health concerns in the World.

For some point in their life, many people struggle with regulating their drinking. Approximately 17 million people aged 18 and older suffer from an alcohol use disorder (AUD), and 1 in 10 children live in a household with a drinking issue parent.

The good news is that no matter how serious the condition can be, most people with a diagnosis of substance use may benefit from some sort of therapy. Evidence reveals that almost one-third of people hospitalized with issues with alcohol do not have any more effects 1 year on. Some people lower their consumption significantly and show less drug related issues. Signs with an alcohol addiction Drug use disorder (AUD) is a psychiatric condition treated by physicians where drinking causes pain or injury to a patient. The diagnosis can vary from moderate to extreme, and is diagnosed with two or three of the following questions when a patient responds "yes."

Have you ever had any moments in the past year that you ended up drinking more, or longer than you intended?

Wanting to cut back or stop drinking more than once, or wanting to, just couldn't? Did you waste any time drinking? And getting ill or seeing the aftereffects overcome? Experienced craving— strong desire to drink, or temptation to? Did you notice that drinking — or getting sick of drinking — always messed with taking care of your family or home? Or caused problems at work? And issues at school? Continued to drink while the relatives or friends were having problems with it? Giving up or cutting down on things that were important or fascinating to you, or having given you pleasure to drink? More than once got into situations that increased your chances of getting hurt (such as driving, swimming, using machinery, walking in a hazardous area or having unsafe sex) while or after you drink?

Continued drinking even if it made you feel depressed or anxious, or added to another health issue? Or after having blackout memory? Would you have had to drink much more than you once had to get the effect you wanted? Or did you think your regular amount of drinks having even less effect than they had before?

Did you notice that you have withdrawal signs while the effects of alcohol were worn off, such as sleep disturbance, shakiness, irritability, agitation, fatigue, restlessness, Nausea or sweating? Or did things which weren't there feel? When you have all of these signs your alcohol might be a source of concern now. The more signs you encounter, the more pressing the need for improvement. A health care practitioner can conduct a formal symptom assessment to see if there is an alcohol-use disorder.

6.3. Primary Care Doctors

Starting with a primary care provider

For someone who cares about diagnosis, going to a primary care doctor is an important first step— he or she may be a reliable source of information and medicines for diagnosis. A primary care physician may also: determine that a patient's drinking behavior is unsafe Help develop a recovery plan Determine mental safety evaluation whether alcohol therapy may be necessary.

6.4. What Medicines are approved by FDA?

Some drugs have been shown to help people interrupt or reduce their alcohol successfully, and prevent relapse.

Registered Drugs Four drugs have been approved by the U.S. Food and Drug Administration (FDA) for treating alcohol dependency, and some are being tested to determine if they are successful.

Naltrexone can help to minimize heavy drinking by humans. Acamprosate makes the prohibition harder to sustain.

Disulfiram inhibits the body's processing of alcohol (metabolism), causing painful effects such as diarrhea, and skin flushing. Those adverse effects can help some people stop taking disulfiram when drinking. This is important to note that not all people can respond to opioids but they can be an effective aid in combating opioid dependency for a subset of individuals.

Scientists are designing a broader variety of prescription therapies that can be adapted to patient needs. If more drugs are affordable, people may be able to try different drugs and figure out which medicines they better respond and.

"Doesn't drugs just swap one addiction for another?"It is not an uncommon problem, but the simple response is' no.' All licensed opioid dependency recovery drugs are non-addictive. Such medications are intended to better treat a chronic illness, just like one would take drugs to keep their asthma or diabetes under control.

Look ahead: The Prospect of Medical Change appears to be made as experts try innovative and improved drug addiction therapies. Through researching the root mechanisms of alcoholism in the brain and body, NIAAA aims to establish specific cellular or molecular properties — considered "targets" — that may contribute to new drug growth.

Personalized medicine

Ideally, health care professionals could identify which treatment for alcoholism is most effective for each individual. The NIAAA and other organizations perform work to determine genes and other factors that can influence how well someone will react to a given treatment. Such developments could improve the manner in which possible care decisions are made.

Present NIAAA Studies — Pointing to Potential Breakthroughs Several medications already licensed for other applications have shown promise to address alcohol dependence and problem drinking: Anti-smoking medication varenicline (marketed as Chantix) has significantly reduced alcohol consumption and cravings among alcoholics.

Gabapentin, a medication used to treat pain conditions and epilepsy, was shown to increase abstinence and reduce heavy drinking. Those taking the medication also reported fewer alcohol cravings and improved mood and sleep. The anti-epileptic topiramate drug has been shown to help people reduce alcohol habits, particularly in those with a certain genetic profile that seems to be related to the efficacy of the therapy.

6.5. Tips for treatment selection

Alcohol recovery experts are providing recommendations on what to expect in seeking a rehab plan. In fact, when making a medical decision, collect as much information as you can about the service or supplier. If you meet someone with first-hand knowledge of the system, inquire about his or her personal experience can be beneficial. Here are some questions that will help direct your choice: What type of care does the plan or service offer?

This is necessary to determine whether the facility is using all the approaches commonly available, or depending on one solution. You will want to know which therapy is provided by the system or service, and whether mental health problems are treated along with alcohol care.

Was therapy personally tailored?

It is crucial for their success that the right treatment is matched to the patient. All would benefit from a particular treatment. Determining how the medication should be adjusted to suit evolving demands when they occur may also be useful.

What is the patient expecting from that?

To determine which treatment best matches your needs, you'll want to consider what will be asked of you.

Was progress calculated in treatment?

You will be able to accurately compare the choices by determining how and how the system or company evaluates the performance.

How is relapse treated by the system or the provider?

Relapse is normal and you'll want to learn how it's being dealt with. See Relapse Is Part of Process for more information on relapse.

While seeking medical assistance, it is crucial that you feel appreciated and heard, and that you have a sense of trust that this individual, community or agency can support. Note, though, that it will take time to establish relationships with physicians, therapists and other health care providers.

6.6. Determining the level of treatment

For several factors, the diagnosis of alcohol use disorders, especially mild or extreme types, may be important. Until the National Institute for Drug Abuse (NIDA) identified depression as "Chronic brain disease," it was considered a biopsychosocial-spiritual disorder. The complicated elements of the term were embraced as it means that all parts of a person's life are influenced by addiction. As health care practitioners, we are always more concerned with our patients ' well-being, rather than the diagnoses ' medical, financial, or spiritual consequences.

Confirmatory clinical tests and test reports will help cut through the frequently resulting withdrawal denial, rationalization, and lack of candor.

Years earlier, "care" with an alcohol or other drug use condition meant that the victim would be whisked away to a remote 28-day rehab center for compliance and modesty to attend intensive lessons. Twenty-eight-day centers of recovery were popularized and spoofed in literature and films. Usage of the 28-day rehabilitation plan for all gravity levels, and all drug usage conditions is focused on justification but not strictly facts.

There is still a role for the 28-day recovery cycle in today's recovery of opioid use disorders, but this continuum of care is often chosen most often based on defined needs-determining requirements.

Current care services are measured and evaluated depending on the seriousness of the condition, the involvement (or absence) of co-occurring illnesses, psychological support and the subject's ability to participate.

Many treatment providers, insurance agencies, and organizations who have developed standards are considered the norm, except those published by the American Society of Addiction Medicine (ASAM). Treatment guidelines for adults and youth are contained in the ASAM Requirements (now 3rd edition). We will be focusing on the adult table for the purposes of this report. The ASAM Patient Placement Criterion uses a numerical method to classify level 4 treatment, which suggests hospital admission as the lowest level of either a medical or therapeutic facility (Figure 1). In Level 4, patients are treated safely in an area where 24-hour health care and emergency facilities are available. Depending on the quality of treatment, examinations, and operations undertaken, the expense of medical facilities will be thousands or hundreds of thousands of dollars a day.

The next lower stage (3.7) makes the use of vital protocols and order sets that help the doctor to prescribe and track care without having to handle the patient as intensively as possible. While facilities that offer 3.7-level services include 24-hour health care, they are also not complete hospitals and provide readily available pharmacy, radiology, and on-call emergency staff at all hours. Tier 3.7 services are less costly than hospital services but costs differ widely based on client base and source of financing.

Rate 3.5 is the "Clinically Managed" high impact treatment. Licensed counselors, social workers, or therapists also offer treatment, with as-needed emergency resources available.

In a supportive care environment or clinical group, the services which have a higher quality level also include providers with a broad range of professional skills. Tier 3.3 is a high intensity rehabilitation care "population-oriented," often with facilities, configuration or variety of programs intended to resolve particular problems (such as neurological impairments). Level 3.1 is deemed residential treatment of low intensity.

This level of care is most often seen as a step-down or intermediate period for people requiring support and a healthy housing atmosphere to sustain the progress achieved at a higher level of service. Many patients continue to work or go to school again when at this stage of care, and collaborate with their recovered friends and clinicians to manage associated stressors.

Treatment centers at level 3.1 also provide financial services to help patients prepare and spend their resources wisely.

Grade 2.5, the most formal treatment in an ambulatory environment is the "Partial Hospitalization Plan." Tier 2.5 services provide daytime care with a clinical low to high intensity program, with the patient returning home at night. Time spent at this point of care is normally more than 20 hours a week. Often known as Comprehensive Outpatient Program (IOP) is stage 2.1 (the next lower step). IOPs have multiple classes or single sessions every day of care and also discuss co-occurring conditions (some have more, others have fewer). Level 2.1's intentional flexibility allows for treatment in the evenings and/or weekends in addition to the usual daytime weekday hours. Time spent at this level in treatment is generally 9-19 hours per week.

Level 1 is ambulatory dependent care, where the doctor and the patient agreeing about the duration of clinic visits. In an office visit environment, patients with co-occurring mental conditions or behavioral issues that may conflict with group dynamics can respond best to individual counseling. Time spent at this point of care is usually less than 9 hours a week. A different classification is Drug Recovery Services (OTPs) with methadone or buprenorphine. With frequent appointments, routine medication tests, and therapy sessions, OTPs can be very formal. They may also be fairly unstructured, with regular drug maintenance office appointments, with no counseling needs.

The lowest level of care is level 0.5 (single office dependent intervention). That degree of care is designed to treat people who do not fit the requirements for a substance misuse or diagnosis of depression but who are considered to be at risk. Patients can be assigned to community treatment services but follow-up appointments to treat drug or other substance misuse are not planned. What care standard to use is based on a 6-dimensional evaluation of the patient's results?

Dimension 1 is signs of alcohol poisoning and/or serious alcohol / other drug withdrawal. Hospitalization is required in patients with serious withdrawal symptoms that need 24 hour medical attention. With less intensive and less costly care choices patients with less serious symptoms can be treated.

The ASAM Criteria contains several tables and maps that measure the level of treatment needed depending on the severity of the effects of withdrawal and the ability to treat withdrawal. Withdrawal control levels correlate to treatment levels, except for level 3.2-WM which applies to all 3.3 and 3.5 treatment levels.

Level 2 is diseases and biomedicine disorders. Patients with severe injury or untreated medical conditions (e.g. malignant hypertension, diabetic ketoacidosis, hyperosmolar non-ketotic hyperglycemia, decompensated cirrhosis, etc.) typically need treatment in the Level 4 environment.

Dimension 3 is the problems and mental, physical, or cognitive disorders. Patients of co-occurring mental, behavioral or neurological conditions that affect the understanding of reality, or others at serious risk of injuring themselves or others need appropriate therapy in an atmosphere that requires all systems to be treated together. Such treatment is also given with one-to - one monitoring in a hospital-based, closed psychiatric unit or emergency clinic.

Area 4 is primed for transition. The keyword that sums this aspect up to the perspective of the authors. The query clinicians would have to inquire about the incentive of the patient to improve. Is the request for treatment more related to avoiding external consequences or a desire to change internally? Ironically, response measurements 4 do not require patients for Tier 4 facilities. It makes sense the doctor isn't the best standard of treatment to provide perspective. This problem is better tackled in a smaller, less intensive standard of treatment, in the absence of Dimension 1, 2, or 3 variables. Dimension 5 is opportunity for relapse, continued use or continued problem. Automaticity is the keyword that sums this element up to the speaker. The participant may be able to relax, understand, and emotionally climb to commitment to improve in a therapy or social session but may instead be unable to avoid drug consumption when faced with previous drinking-related signs or stressors. Inability to resist impulse is not a cause for hospitalization, although in some situations (depending on severity) can prohibit the use of ambulatory care environments.

Dimension 6 is an environment for recuperation. This scale is Dimension 5 is closely related in that a lonely or unsupportive environment can exert pressure on the patient to return to the same mechanism of escape (alcohol, other drugs or behaviors) used before treatment intervention. The benefits of a positive rehabilitation atmosphere cannot be overestimated as an unsafe environment which promotes relapse will easily undo therapy gains. Participating in sobriety meetings and/or developing a network of sober accountability partners and friends can sometimes build a safe environment. Some times more extreme interventions are required, such as removing the patient from a dangerous environment, or exposing friends and/or family members to toxic factors.

6.7. Case Example

Initial Diagnosis

A 64y / o man voluntarily show tremulous and distressed with a blood alcohol content of 320 mg / dl in emergency room.

It is noted that he has a blood pressure of 210/120 mmHg and has a heartbeat of 120 Beats per Minute. He laments nausea on his arms and legs, and diarrhea, pain, and a prickly feeling.

He is asleep, disheveled, and odourless. Funduscopic, respiratory, lung, and abdominal tests are common. CBC and the chemistry panel are regular, and a test for urinary toxicology is pending. Consultation on recovery is called upon to assist with effective diagnosis and temperament. Which care level does the patient need?

Care Recommendations

The condition is now needing Level 4 care. His high pulse and blood pressure along with diarrhea make him inadequate for lower treatment. He can be put on a detoxification regimen activated treatment or symptom, and given as required fluids, thiamine, antinausea, and antihypertensives.

History

The following day, though he still feels tremulous and nervous, the patient is feeling much better. He appears to experience headaches and the feeling of prickly skin, but nausea is worsening, and no vomiting happened overnight. The BP is actually 140/80 mm Hg, and the rhythm is 96 bpm. The patient is able to share the story now. Since his childhood years he has been using alcohol, and has never had any prior therapy for addiction. Since graduating he married his college sweetheart.

He'd be binge drinking weekends during his 20s while enjoying games with his buddies. He enjoyed wine sampling during his 30s, and would share a bottle of wine with friends every night while still binge drinking on weekends. His job promotions during his 40s and 50s provided for business lunches with alcohol use. Before going home and drinking wine before, during and after dinner, he started meeting clients and co-workers after work for drinks. After getting home for the evening, he would go out with "bar mates" but lost interest in any previously enjoyable things (movies, evening walks, sex) He started having complaints over his heavy drinking with his mom, and dull lifestyle. At age 62, he withdrew from work and remained at home for several days, beginning his morning drinking with mimosas and continuing to do it all day. Fights worsened with his mom. He violently attacked his wife during an argument, just three weeks before entry. She called the police who took him out of his room. She replaced the locks, locked the windows and doors and mounted an alarm system. She accuses him of domestic violence, has demanded a restraining order and has not ever spoken to him. He's been living and drinking non-stop with his "Bar buddies" He realizes that he needs to adjust but he doesn't know how. His wife is very angry. What's next step for him in treatment?

<u>**Diagnosis and Treatment Plan**</u>

He has type 1 alcohol use disorder as manifested by multiple negative consequences (struggles with spouse including legal domestic violence intervention), tolerance, and symptoms of withdrawal. He needs to get away from its implications but he is unsure about his internal drive to improve (angry at wife).

His automaticity is unknown, but the environment for his recovery is dangerous. The goal is to finish detoxification and resolve the residual medical problems, and then move him to a rehabilitation rehab center (3.3 or 3.5) based on what his health provider wants to provide.

<u>**Follow-up**</u>

The patient returns after a month in a therapeutic care center of mild duration (level 3.3). He has enjoyed the group attendance and recuperation activities. He no longer shows the urge to drink alcohol, and is not discouraged while visiting the grocery store or restaurant. He knows he's hurting his mom and wants to make amends. He left Alcoholic Anonymous (AA) and then got sponsor. He wants to spend another month of recovery because he doesn't want to return to life with his "Bar friends." The clinic approached his wife who is happy with the prospect of marriage, but "Not yet." What is his next step in treatment?

<u>**Assessment and Strategy**</u>

He developed experience and does not mention automaticity issues. His biggest concern is Dimension 6 — the risky climate for healing. He may make the transition to the lower 3.1 care stage. Now that he understands his role in damaging his marriage, exploring involving the wife in their own recovery program may be possible. When all heal, there is hope for ambulatory pair therapy and reconciliation.

6.8. Other Pharmacological intervention

The problems of inadequate adherence and moderate efficacy with the new FDA-approved medicines prompted the hunt for other options. Among the drugs under investigation are topiramate, baclofen, ondansetron, sertraline, nalmefene, aripiprazole, zonisamide, quetiapine, varenicline and levetiracetamare. Topiramate is known to act as a GABA agonist and antagonist of glutamate.

Topiramate was found to have a lower number of heavy drinking days (N= 371) by participants in a randomized controlled trial than placebo (by 16 percent).In the test, participants randomized to topiramate were titrated from a starting dose of 25mg / day to 300mg / day over a 6-to 8-week span.

Adverse effects that included paresthesia, perversion of taste, and anorexia were troublesome. Certain studies have also demonstrated substantial gain in piramate-using topics of study. While not approved by the FDA for this reason, piramate is considered by some as a first-line treatment choice for alcohol use disorder. Baclofen is reportedly under review as an agonist of GABAB.

A longitudinal open-label research assessed the proportions of high-risk drinkers who were either abstinent or intoxicated at moderate rates one year after start of high-dose baclofen treatment (129 + 71 mg / day). The investigators have been able to track 132 out of 181 cases. 80 per cent of the patients were either abstinent or low-level smoking. Ondansetron is a serotonin type 3 receptor antagonist (5-HT3), which has been approved for nausea which vomiting therapy.

One research randomized 283 alcohol-dependent patients via serotonin transporter (5-HTT) genotype (LL, LS, SS), with additional transporter polymorphism (TT / TG / GG) genotyping. Participants either got twice daily ondansetron 4 µg / kg, or placebo for 11 weeks plus CBT.

The investigators noticed that people with the LL genotype had a lower mean number of drinks a day, and a higher proportion of abstinent days than those consuming placebo, with the largest influence being the LL / TT genotypes of people.

 Sertraline, a selective serotonin synthesis inhibitor licensed to treat depression, anxiety and other psychological conditions, has also been tested for possible efficacy in alcohol-use conditions. One research assessed the impact of sertraline on alcohol-dependent patients, distinguishing them by phenotype (late onset / low vulnerability [LOA] vs early onset / high vulnerability [EOA]) and genotype (LL, LS, SS) serotonin transporter (5-HTT)

 During the 12-week study, the patients (N= 134) were randomised to receive up to 200 mg of sertraline or placebo daily. The influence of the drug differed greatly by both phenotype and genotype, with patients with LOA / LL recording several days of drinking and heavy drinking. Participants in the study were followed only for 6 months post-treatment with ongoing substantially beneficial outcomes for the LOA / LL community. In a randomized double-blind sample in Finland the opioid blocker nalmefene was evaluated.

For the 28-week test, participants (N= 242) took 10 to 40 mg of nalmefene or placebo with limited psychosocial reaction. With 57 participants in the nalmefene arm who were then randomized to either start nalmefene or get placebo, the analysis was extended by 24 weeks.

In both steps, the analysis demonstrated considerably diminished consumption for those receiving nalmefene over placebo. Aripiprazole is an atypical antipsychotic drug often licensed for treatment of bipolar disorder, autism, autistic disorder-related irritability and Tourette syndrome. This is a selective agonist of the receptors Dopamine2 (D2) and serotonin 1A (5-HT1A), and serotonin 2A (5-HT2A) receptor antagonist. For one test, non-treatment-seeking alcohol dependent subjects were randomized to either aripiprazole or placebo, with the dosage titrated up to 15 mg over a 14-day period. During sensitivity to alcohol dependent signs, functional magnetic resonance imaging (MRI) was performed.

In the right ventral striatum of people receiving placebo, brain activation was weaker, and blunted in those receiving aripiprazole. During the 14 day period, patients diagnosed with aripiprazole have had slightly less alcohol drinking. Zonisamide, first synthesized in Japan in the 1970s, is an anticonvulsant drug licensed as an adjunctive medication for the treatment of intermittent epileptic seizures in adults. It is chemically known as sulfonamide, acts to block voltage-dependent sodium and calcium channels, and is metabolized mainly by 3A4 (CYP3A4) liver cytochrome. In a double-blind trial, 40 people with alcohol use disorder were randomized to undergo combination zonisamide (up to 500 mg / d) and 12 weeks of psychosocial or placebo treatment or psychosocial counseling.

While there was no statistically meaningful gap in abstinent days between classes, there was a substantial decrease in heavy-drinking days per week. Varenicline, an FDA-approved medication for the treatment of nicotine dependency, was shown at a dosage of 2mg / day to substantially minimize heavy drinking days a week, drinks a day and alcohol cravings in smokers and non-smokers Complementary and Alternative Medicine (CAM) The patient may find it daunting to qualify for medication with an opioid use problem.

Individuals have a strong propensity to ask if there is maybe an simpler or cheaper choice before taking the decision to take the initial, most daunting path into recovery.

Addiction medication complementary and alternative medications (CAMs) are available internationally, and have gained popularity in the United States. It will be a complicated task to define and explain the large variety of available CAMs. In this context, even the concept of CAM is difficult as behavioural therapy, 12-step support groups, and stress relief / relaxation techniques are all part of existing non-alternative recovery programs.

Founded in 1998, the National Center for Holistic and Integrative Health (NCCIH), previously known as the National Center for Complementary and Alternative Medicine (NCCAM), is one of 27 centers that make up the National Institute for Safety. Their Strategic Strategy for 2016 identifies the following targets:

1. Advance the advancement of basic research and technology

2. Boost treatment for conditions which are difficult to treat

3. Promoting hygiene, and avoiding disease

4. Enhance workplace for effective and equitable wellness study

5. Disseminate comprehensive evidence-based knowledge on holistic and integrative wellness treatments. These approaches may be effective in experiments using biofeedback and electroacupuncture.

There is a lack of randomized, placebo / sham controlled studies that use those therapies. Nonetheless, it is important to stress that lack of evidence is separate from lack of effectiveness. Individuals who conquered their fights with alcohol using CAM have shared several testimonials of performance. In fact, firms with patented formulas or treatments used testimony as a marketing tactic to sell CAM products directly to the consumers. It is difficult to assess or compare the possible value of these therapies, since they have still not received the thorough review needed for introduction or publishing in scientific meetings or journals.

Chapter 7: Famous Personalities Who Recovered from Alcoholism

An estimated 16 million adults in the U.S. had an alcohol use disorder, or alcoholism, in 2015. This is a severe, persistent epidemic that can affect everyone, including celebrities in Hollywood.

Because of the lifestyle and strain, famous people, particularly young ones, maybe at an increased risk of drug and alcohol addiction. Many stars have surmounted their alcoholism, while some are either dealing with it or have even died. A few are listed below.

Zac Efron

Zac Efron Efron, the former teenage star of High School Musical, recently talked about his battle with drugs and alcoholism. After a high-profile trip to recovery, Efron continued to go on drinking and even hurt himself so badly in a fall that doctors had to weld his jaw shut. Still, now, Efron lives a healthy lifestyle. He left Associated Alcoholics (AA) and is seeing a therapist. He tells the Hollywood Reporter that addiction is "a relentless struggle."2 Amy Winehouse, a five-time winner of the Grammy Award, is known for songs such as" Rehab, "which feature lyrics about avoiding drug and alcohol abuse care. During the last years of her life,

Winehouse openly suffered from alcoholism and drug addiction, and her image as a party girl quickly overshadowed her talents as a singer. Like most famous alcoholics, her health rapidly declined. She died from alcohol poisoning in 2011, at the age of 27.

Bradley Cooper

Bradley Cooper is well known for his roles in a comedy film. But like most of us, there have been ups and downs in Cooper's life. He is a recoverer from alcoholism and has been sober for more than ten years. In 2015, he explained how alcohol had influenced practically everything in his life, "if I hadn't changed my life, I wouldn't have had access to myself or other people, or even have been able to take in other people. I'd never have had the relationships I'm doing. I would never have been able to look after my father the way I did when he was sick. Too many things. "The comments from Cooper point to the fact that alcohol affects more than just you — it often affects those around you.

Daniel Radcliffe

Like many other child actors, the beloved star of the "Harry Potter" series has struggled to grow up in show business. Although Harry's character was innocent and noble, he was influenced by real-life struggles for Daniel Radcliffe, namely his alcohol addiction. In an interview published in ShortListmagazine in 2012, Radcliffe mentioned how he discovered that "drinking was toxic and detrimental to my body and my social life," and how he had become "a 20-year-old recluse." He also revealed how he used to drink before going on the set, and how he respected Gary Oldman, a co-star who would also be addicted to alcohol.

Radcliffe acknowledges, despite being sober, that maintaining his sobriety at events where there is alcohol is not straightforward. Some of the best lessons he has learned are that he would have allowed himself to have a sober life. In the same interview, he said, "I had to interrupt myself. And stopping showed me a world of joy that I didn't think was possible. "It is a lesson from Radcliffe that we should all know.

Carrie Fisher

Aside from her popularity in "Star Wars" as Princess Leia, Carrie Fisher was also noted for her public comments about her health and addictions. These included ghosts. She also wrote a book about her struggles in 2008, entitled "Wishful Drinking." She writes in the book, "Happy is one of many things that I'm likely to be in a day and definitely during a lifetime. Yet I think if you want to be satisfied in your life — more to the point, if you need to feel relaxed all the time —

then, among other things, you have the makeup of a typical drug addict or alcoholic. "Yes, alcohol is sometimes used as a coping strategy, and Fisher explains — in her usual humorous way — how to make it worse.

Tragically, in December 2016, Fisher died from a heart attack. A relapse is believed to have been partly to blame. Fans are also grieving the absence of the endearing star.

Billy Joel Popular pop / rock singer

Billy Joel has admitted in his adult life to struggling with drug abuse. Apparently, alcohol got in the way of his job and personal connections. Fellow musician (and sometimes touring partner) Elton John begged Joel to seek alcohol treatment. John is quoted in an early 2011 issue of Rolling Stone as saying that Joel wanted to check into "tough" therapy, and that drinking was getting in the way of his life and career.

Joel muses on his past drinking habits in a 2013 interview with The New York Times Magazine: "I don't know why I drank so much that I don't subscribe to A.A., I don't subscribe to the 12-step things. Occasionally I just overdid it ... but it wasn't regular, it would be periods of time, during a divorce or something. "Even if drinking wasn't regular, this is another form of alcohol addiction identified by binge-drinking Joel.

Stephen King

World-famous horror author Stephen King suffered for a long period with drugs and alcohol. King's family and associates orchestrated an intervention in 1987, throwing evidence before him of his addictions. In the late 1980s King sought immediate help and quit all forms of drugs and alcohol.

King opened up his former drug abuse to The Guardian in 2013, explaining how he is not shamed by his history. He said, "There's one thing in AA, which they're reading in a lot of meetings, 'The Promises.' Some of those promises have come true in my life, that's real, we're going to come to know a new freedom and new joy. Yet it also says in there, "We're not going to mourn the past, nor want to close the door on it. And on the past, I have no wish to close the door. I was pretty honest on my history. Still I regret it? I do. I do. I do. I do. I regret the need. "King's not going to say that he hasn't had any problems with alcohol, nor does he think he can hide it. It's a part of who he is and since his family intervention, he has been sober.

Robin Williams

The popular comedian abused cocaine and alcohol early in his career but left when his friend and fellow comedian, John Belushi, died in 1982 from an overdose of cocaine and heroin.

The late star then battled off and on with alcohol for years before his death in 2014. Such challenges he also frequently highlighted as part of his stand-up routines. Williams talked about the fact in a 2006 interview with Diane Sawyer that alcohol doesn't always have a motive behind it, saying "It's [addiction]—not induced by anything, it's just there," Williams said. "Waiting. It's waiting for the moment you think, 'It's all right now, I'm all right.' Suddenly, the next thing you know, it's not all right. You realize then, "Where am I? I didn't know that I was in Cleveland. '"Williams sadly died in 2014. Just before his death he was confirmed to have just entered Rehab again.

Betty Ford

Betty Ford, former President Gerald Ford's wife, suffered from alcoholism and painkiller addiction. Through confessing to her longstanding struggle with alcoholism in the 1970s, she increased public consciousness of addiction. Once she eventually recovered, the Betty Ford Center was formed to help people tackle drug and alcohol abuse.

Perhaps Ford's biggest achievement was the sincerity that she brought to the notion of alcoholism in America. Anybody may get addicted to alcohol. She was quoted as saying "My makeup wasn't smeared, I wasn't disheveled, I acted socially, and I never finished a bottle so how could I be alcoholic? "In other words, alcoholism does not show stereotypical symptoms. Even being the first US lady doesn't make you prone to alcoholism.

Mel Gibson

For all of his adult life, Mel Gibson has openly admitted fighting alcoholism. He was arrested for driving under the influence in 2009. During a previous arrest during 2006, made on suspicion of drunk driving, the arresting officer alleged he made antisemitic remarks. Gibson sought medical treatment in the past, and for his drug addiction, he checked himself into Rehab.

The Fix reported Gibson set out the harsh truth that comes with dreaming about leaving alcohol in 2016. "They say there are only three options: you're going crazy, you're going to die, or you're going to leave." ADVERTISEMENT Get answers from a doctor in minutes, do you have any medical questions? Talk online or over the phone with a board-certified, professional doctor. Pediatrists and other professionals are on hand 24/7.

Lindsay Lohan

Like other teen stars, the young starlet has discussed drug and alcohol abuse in public. Lohan has to work hard to remain sober, and in 2011 one unsuccessful attempt at a recovery has already been made. She was required to wear an alcohol screening bracelet by court order in 2010 to control her alcohol intake. Lohan had a public relapse on her reality show in 2014, showing how to beat alcohol addiction is an ongoing battle truly.

Lohan was honest about other dangers that alcohol might pose, too. Lohan said in an interview with Oprah Winfrey in 2013 that alcohol "was for me a gateway to other things ... I tried cocaine with alcohol."

David Hasselhoff

David Hasselhoff became notorious for his alcoholism because of his starring role on "Baywatch." In 2007, a home video from a drunken Hasselhoff went viral, receiving airtime on countless news programs and the internet. His rights to visitation with his daughters were briefly revoked, and he was forced to seek medical treatment for his addiction.

He told the Mirror in 2015 "It is my job to do the best I can and to take things one day at a time. Yet alcohol can turn deadly. The most disgusting thing is when you go into a meeting, and you're like, 'Where is Steve? 'And they say,' Last night, Oh Steve died. But you saw him just yesterday! It's a very frightening, dangerous thing that needs to be tackled.

"However, in these days, Hasselhoff takes his struggles with alcohol even more seriously and has also chosen to change his lifestyle with diet and exercise fully.

Conclusion

The cause of disorder related to alcohol use is still unknown. Disorder of alcohol use develops when you are drinking so much that there are chemical changes in the brain. Such improvements improve the pleasurable feelings when you drink alcohol. That makes you want to drink more frequently, even if it does harm.

The pleasurable feelings associated with alcohol use eventually go away, and the person with alcohol use disorder will engage in drinking to prevent symptoms of withdrawal. These can be quite unpleasant and even dangerous withdrawal symptoms.

Traditionally, alcohol use disorder develops gradually over time. Running inside families is also popular. While the exact cause of alcohol use disorder is unclear, there are some factors that may increase your risk of developing this disease.

Known risk factors include having: more than 15 drinks per week if you are male than 12 drinks per week if you are female more than 5 drinks per day at least once a week (binge drinking) a mental health disorder parent with alcohol use disorder, such as depression, anxiety, or schizophrenia You may also be at a higher risk of alcohol use disorder if you: are a young adult with a peer experience.

This book has tried to throw light on every social, medical and psychological aspect of alcoholism.